BALD IS BETTER

WITH EARRINGS

BALD IS BETTER
WITH EARRINGS

A Survivor's Guide to Getting
Through Breast Cancer

ANDREA
HUTTON

HARPER WAVE

An Imprint of HarperCollins*Publishers*

This book is written as a source of information only. The information contained in this book should by no means be considered a substitute for the advice of a qualified medical professional, who should always be consulted before beginning any new diet, exercise, or other health program. All efforts have been made to ensure the accuracy of the information contained in this book as of the date published. The author and the publisher expressly disclaim responsibility for any adverse effects arising from the use or application of the information contained herein.

HarperCollins books may be purchased for educational, business, or sales promotional use. For information, please e-mail the Special Markets Department at SPsales@harpercollins.com.

FIRST EDITION

Design by Fritz Metsch

Library of Congress Cataloging-in-Publication Data has been applied for.

ISBN: 978-0-06-237565-0

15 16 17 18 19   OV/RRD   10 9 8 7 6 5 4 3 2 1

This book is dedicated
to my family and friends.

Especially:

Richard, my wonderful husband, for loving and supporting me in sickness and in health, and without whom there would be no book.

Jeremy and Marisa, my incredible children, who are the most amazing young adults and who make me proud every single day.

Alan and Carol, my loving parents, who have always been there to care for and support me.

Old friends in Seattle who came to chemo, cooked, and walked with me.

New friends in California who, thankfully, do not have to do any of those things but still choose to walk with me.

To those who are now unfortunate enough to need this book—I hope you find something here to help you, comfort you, and give you hope.

CONTENTS

Contents

Contents

INTRODUCTION

∽

Labor Day weekend 2009. The beginning of the rest of my life. The weekend I crossed the street from normal to Cancer Girl . . . and then, thankfully, to survivor. The next year would be filled with the pain, scars, fears, needle pricks, tests, results, hair losses and gains, weight losses and gains, sleep deprivation, fatigue, drug reactions and interactions, and the million and one other experiences that would challenge, exhaust, and exhilarate me and everyone in my family and circle of friends.

I wish this were a singular experience, but it is one shared by millions of women around the world. Whether it's an epidemic or not, breast cancer is a part of every woman's life. If you don't have it, you fear it. From the mammograms designed to detect it, to the walks and ribbons raising money to stop it, we are inundated by *breast cancer awareness.*

I don't care how aware you might be—a diagnosis

throws you into a tailspin so fast you lose your bearings, breath, and possibly a breast or two.

With two teenage kids, a few moves around the country, and various job experiences, I figured I was pretty well equipped to handle just about anything life could throw at me. Boy, was I ever wrong! There's nothing like being diagnosed with a life-threatening illness to remind you that you are just a collection of cells and moving parts that can turn against you at any time. I thought losing those pesky twenty pounds and raising two kids were tough. What was I thinking? With breast cancer, losing the weight was easy— nothing like a little chemo diet to get you started.

When I was diagnosed, I wanted to know everything. I educated myself as much as possible. I read every book, article, and Web site I could find and talked to everyone I knew, but nothing would prepare me for the experiences of surgery, chemotherapy, and radiation. Part of the problem was that I wanted to know what everything would *feel* like. What tricks could I use to ease my pain and discomfort? Was I the only one who felt certain things? What did they mean by "fatigue?" When *exactly* would my hair fall out, and how? I wanted a guide—a how-to for the Cancer Girl I had become.

For me, at least, there just wasn't enough of the

right kind of information out there. I didn't care what the normal breast looked like and how the cell walls of tumors were constructed. I really wasn't interested in all the biology—I wanted to know what to expect after surgery when I looked at my mastectomy scar. I wanted to know how to begin to come to terms with this diagnosis, and what the treatments would really mean for me and my family. I wanted to know how bad the nausea would really be, what it would feel and look like to be bald, and what I could possibly do to help myself feel better during this awful time in my life. So I asked a million questions, kept notes, and wrote a blog along the way so I could, perhaps, write it down for others—maybe offer some small help to the next woman who would hear those horrific words: "It's cancer."

This is not a medical text. You will not find descriptions of breast tissue or the chemical components of chemotherapy drugs. You will not find every single question answered or every experience covered. Your journey is your own, and nobody will have the exact same one. I cannot tell you how you got here or where you're going next. However, this book is, quite simply, the book I tried to find when I was diagnosed. A plain and straightforward (and hopefully sometimes funny and uplifting) how-to for a few of the situations you may find yourself in now that you've heard those scary words: "You've got breast cancer." This is just one of many resources that may keep you from getting run over by a bus as you cross the street to my side.

HOW TO READ THIS BOOK

Now that you've been diagnosed, you'll want to know what to expect. I'll tell you about the tests, the chemo, shaving your head, being bald, the radiation, the emotional and physical roller coaster you've stepped onto, in roughly the order that things happened to me—the diagnosis, the tests, surgery, chemo, radiation, and everything that comes after. You can go to the Contents page and read just the parts that relate to what's happening to you in real time. The tricks for surviving chemo. How to keep your skin from crisping during radiation. How to keep track of your meds, and so on. Or you can read the whole book from start to finish. I wrote this book to be your BCCB—breast cancer companion book. I hope it provides some answers, solace, and even a chuckle or two.

BALD IS BETTER

WITH EARRINGS

My Story

THE LUMPS

On Thursday, August 20 I felt a lump in my right breast. I'd found a bunch of weird things over the years that resolved after I got my period or were gone the next day. This one felt different. I called my doctor, who examined me and assured me it was just a cyst. I was forty-one years old with no risk factors for breast cancer, so we didn't think much of it. It felt round and solid, the size of a soybean. I kept touching it. The only thing that made me nervous was that it was a little painful. I searched the Internet for clues, and it certainly seemed most likely to be a cyst. I had a regular mammogram scheduled in a few weeks, but my doctor decided to set up a diagnostic mammogram sooner, on Friday, August 28.

I learned my most important lesson that day: Never go to a mammogram alone. You need a bosom buddy. I tell everyone to *always* have someone go with them, because *this* is where you find out you might have cancer. It's in the way the nurse will let you know the doctor would like more pictures. It's in the way she changes from bubbly and cheerful to quietly efficient as you go back for more images.

After an excruciating mammogram, I went back to the waiting room while they checked the results. Then the technician came to tell me the doctor needed more pictures—that is, more uncomfortable squashing. Then back to the waiting room. The technician reappeared and whispered in my ear that the radiologist wanted to do an ultrasound.

This is where your heart drops to the floor. I went back to the examining room and lay down. A nurse and the radiologist started the ultrasound, and I could tell immediately I had cancer by the way they were pointing at the screen and being oh-so careful not to show anything on their faces. I was lying on the table thinking, Oh my God, I have cancer. I can't believe this. And I'm not saying anything because they're not saying anything. Until finally I can't take it anymore, and I say, "Obviously it's not good, so when are you going to tell me?" The radiologist says, "Let's not get ahead of ourselves. We need to look at a few more things." Sure, right. Did you guys not see the elephant that just walked into the room? A big, scary elephant with the word "cancer" written all over it? And they continue the ultrasound, pointing and measuring and clicking while my heart is pounding in my chest, and I'm trying to be calm because I want to be smart and aware and not pass out. Then they're finished and they ask me whether anyone is with me. Like I said, not good.

So, never, *ever* go to your mammogram alone. In fact, starting now, don't go to *any* doctors alone if you can help it. Obviously you can't always have someone with you, but it's really helpful when someone else is there. Sometimes there's just so much information that it's great to have another set of ears in the room—particularly if they can take notes for you to look at later.

I was lucky that my husband, Richard, had decided to come with me when I went for my mammogram. I wasn't even sure why he'd wanted to come, to be honest, but later he told me that when he felt the lump, he was worried, so he thought he'd better be there. So they bring him in, and I'm sitting up now in my gown, kind of shaking, and he holds on to me, and the doctor says that he's going to say some things, and we'll probably forget almost everything we hear. My husband says, "Oh no we won't." The doctor looks at us sympathetically and says there are actually two lumps in my right breast, and we won't know for sure unless they do a core biopsy, but there's cause for concern. Now I'm shaking like a leaf, but I am completely aware of everything that he's saying. In fact I say, "Ignore the fact that I'm shaking. I understand everything you're saying." My husband is holding my shoulders, and we're staring at each other, and we're listening while he tells us they can do the biopsy now, or we can wait and make an appointment with a breast surgeon and then they'll order it. We agree that there's no time to waste—we're assuming it's cancer, right? The sooner you start doing stuff, the better.

So they numb my breast as best they can, and then they stick in this giant needle with a kind of sucking thing on it, and they dig it deep into my breast, because that's where the lumps are, and it hurts like hell. They keep telling me they're sorry that it hurts, but it's really deep. And my husband is standing outside now, because this is not something he should see, and when they ask him to come back, I've got an ice pack on my boob, and I'm really shaking. They give us business cards for two breast surgeons and tell us we should call them on Monday. Of course it's Friday evening now. We walk out of the office stunned, a little numb, and I'm in serious pain.

We keep saying, "Let's not get ahead of ourselves.

We won't know anything for sure until we get the re-sults," but it was just so obvious from the way they were talking that it wasn't going to be good news. I was shocked. Floored actually. I mean, I was forty-one and had no risk factors. My grandmother had died of breast cancer at seventy-six, but every doctor told me that didn't count. My mother was fine, and I was forty-one! I didn't smoke, I had breast-fed my kids, I wasn't overweight, I ate well, I exercised. Sure, I was a chocoholic and probably drank too much Diet Coke, but breast cancer? No way!

One of my friends knew I was having a mammo-gram and got nervous when I didn't call her back af-ter a few hours. She assumed the worst and called her neighbor, who happened to be an excellent oncologist. She told my friend I should call her in the morning. She turned out to be a lifesaver—literally.

So now it's Friday evening, and we're pretty sure I have breast cancer. The nurse and radiologist just looked so severe and serious it was hard to imagine it was going to be good news. We don't say anything to our teenage kids, because we don't know what to say, and we try to figure out what comes next. Who do we know? How do we find the right surgeon? What do we do first? I call the oncologist the next day and tell her what happened. She tells me it sounds like I'm not going to get good news, but this is a treatable disease and you have to take one step at a time.

This becomes a recurring theme. You will hear this over and over: Take one day at a time. Don't get ahead of yourself. Try to focus on the present. It's great advice, but certainly in those first few days and weeks, absolutely impossible to follow. You will learn how. You will find that as things go on, it's easier to do. Not every day—but some days.

In this book I'm going to tell you what I know from experience and from interviewing other women, nurses, and doctors. I'm going to give it to you straight and offer as much practical information and advice as I can. At the end of each section you'll find my Top 5 lists. These are the five things I think are vital to remember each step of the way. Here's my first Top 5, which is critical right now, almost immediately after you've heard the news:

TOP 5 TIPS FOR WHEN YOU ARE FIRST DIAGNOSED

∞

1. Don't panic. Well, you can panic a little, but not so much that you can't function.

---

2. Rally the troops. Think of anyone you know who might be able to help you navigate the next steps.

3. Breathe. This is just the beginning. You don't know much yet. Next come the tests and more tests. You can do this.

4. Stay away from the Internet. This is not the time to start researching everything that's ever been posted about breast cancer and all the statistics. The statistics are scary, and they don't apply to you yet. You don't know anything yet. Actually, this is good advice for the whole of your treatment: Stay away from random chat boards on the subject. They can freak you out unnecessarily.

5. Don't panic. Yup, worth saying again.

2

Tests

The next doctor you'll be referred to is either a surgeon or a medical oncologist. In most cases it will be a surgeon. This will be fine by you because right about now you're probably just thinking, *Get it out!* Also, having an appointment with a medical oncologist before they have all the information that comes with surgery (type and size of tumor, positive or negative sentinel nodes, and so on) can be a little overwhelming, because without the lab results from surgery or biopsy it will be hard for them to prescribe the next step in treatment.

Regardless of whether you start with an oncologist or a breast surgeon—and I started with an oncologist, because that's whom I found first—after the core biopsies come the tests, and the waiting for results, and the question marks followed by more tests. Meanwhile, all you can think is—Just get it *out* already! I have cancer, and it's growing every day. Isn't it more likely to spread every day that I wait? The truth is that most breast cancers grow quite slowly, and the few days or weeks it takes to get all the tests done and everything scheduled don't increase the chances that it's spreading, but it is sure hard to sleep!

Let me say it now, and I'll repeat it later: The tests and the waiting are endless. This doesn't change. Ever. Once you've entered the Cancer Club, every visit starts with the waiting room. And no matter how little fun you're having, and how relieved you are to leave, it always takes too long to schedule the next visit, the next test, and it takes even longer to get the results. Or that's what it feels like, anyway.

I suggest you bring something to keep you busy while you're waiting; whether it's a friend or loved one who can help you pass the time, work, or a book that you love, you're going to need something to help distract you from the whirling thoughts in your head. Do not rely on the waiting room magazines. The usual selection is more *Living with Cancer* than the latest *People*.

One of the things you'll have to think about is whom you should tell and how soon. I'll talk about that later. My husband and I chose not to say anything to anyone right away. We wanted to know what we were dealing with first.

MRI

Most likely your next test following the biopsy will be a breast MRI. Depending on where you live and what the scheduling is like, this can take anywhere from a day to a week or so to schedule. The MRI is used to determine how large the cancer is, whether there are any abnormal sites in the other breast, and also if there are any enlarged lymph nodes in the armpit that may signify that the cancer has spread.

An MRI uses a powerful magnetic field, radio frequency pulses, and a computer to produce detailed pictures of organs, soft tissues, bone, and virtually all other internal body structures. The images will then be examined on a computer monitor by a radiologist, and the results sent to your doctor. You can, and should, also have the images copied onto a CD that you take with you and keep in your records.

It wasn't my first MRI. I'd had ankle problems, and I'd been in the tube with all the knocking and clanging before. This one is different. First of all, when they were looking at my ankle, it wasn't a life-or-death situation. I wasn't lying there thinking about what it might mean. This MRI starts the same way. You go into the changing room and take off any and all metal you might be wearing, put on a gown, leave your stuff in a locker, and walk into the testing room, which they have to keep freezing cold because of the machine. That's where the similarities end.

The weirdest thing about a breast MRI is that you lie facedown, and there are these cups for your breasts. At least it doesn't hurt. You just lie there with your boobs hanging down for a while. I kept thinking of that song, "Let your boobs hang low, let them wobble to and fro . . . let your boobs hang low." You've got to do something to avoid thinking about the results of this test. Sing (silently). Dance (in your head). Recite the Declaration of Independence. Do anything you can think of to distract yourself from the what-ifs. You'll need this advice for the multiple tests you'll be having for years to come.

The radiologists look at both breasts and your lymph nodes to see if anything lights up. Based on what they see in an MRI, they may order further testing. If they think there may be lymph node involvement, they'll order other tests. Including more biopsies. Yup, more needles.

I had a lymph biopsy after my MRI. It meant they were worried that the cancer (which, by the way, they hadn't yet told me was cancer) had spread. For me, at least, it wasn't as painful as the breast core biopsy, although it's the same process, this time under my arm. First they stick a needle in the area and shoot lidocaine in to numb it. Then they stick in that same kind of suction needle device they used in the first lump biopsy while the nurse shows them where to go with the ultrasound. They say that thing you know is code: "You're going to feel some pressure." It's code for "pain." The sensation is definitely pressure. Lots of pressure. In your armpit. This happens a few times. There's lots of talking between the doctor and the nurse, and everyone is nice and also matter-of-fact. Still—big, painted-pink, ribbon-wearing cancer elephant in the room. Talk about *stress*!

TOP 5 TIPS FOR YOUR FIRST MRI

∞

1. Ask for a copy of the scan when you check in, and tell them you'd like to take it with you. This advice goes beyond all your scans. It's incredibly important that you have a comprehensive set of your

own records. You might have to change doctors or hospitals—or sometimes even the most reliable office can misplace things. And you (and everyone around you) will forget things. Always, always keep a copy of all your own records.

2. Have someone you trust bring you to the test and take you home. It can be emotionally draining as well as physically taxing.

3. Make sure to take off anything metal. Jewelry, zippers, anything. And take off your shoes, even though they may tell you that you don't have to. One time I left my flats on, and when they began to move me into the machine, my feet started to be pulled up toward my chest. I almost had to yell for them to stop. There must have been metal inside the little heels on my shoes.

4. Relax. After this you'll still have to wait for the doctor's appointment before you get the results.

5. Ice is your friend. Use it. Biopsy needles are invasive, and they can damage the tissues they pass through. Ice reduces swelling. After any biopsy, as soon as you get home, apply ice—twenty minutes on, twenty minutes off for an hour, and then again after a few

> hours if it still hurts. Remember always to cover the ice pack with something. Do not apply it directly to the skin. Take ibuprofen if the site is sore.

PET SCAN

I call this the "PREP" scan because there's a lot you have to do to prepare for it. Officially, though, it is a Positron-Emission Tomography/Computed Tomography (PET/CT) scan. It is used to produce images that pinpoint the location of abnormal metabolic activity within the body. First you will probably be asked to follow dietary restrictions for a day or so, depriving yourself of sugar and carbohydrates for twenty-four hours. This is because cancer cells grow quickly and require a lot of glucose. Limiting your intake of glucose before the test allows the scanner to detect any cells that are emitting signs of high glucose use when you're administered glucose during the test. Then you have to drink two huge bottles of this liquid, which is a type of barium "milk." Notice the quotation marks. It looks milk-like, but it's actually chalk-like. Usually you drink one at home and one at the test center. It's no big deal. And it's really not that bad. Mocha is one choice, but don't be fooled: It's not your usual from Starbucks. I've had quite a few scans, and I've tasted all but banana. Mocha is the best—of course that's not saying much. I recommend using a straw to drink the stuff. It makes it go down a little easier.

This is the only test with audience participation. Every doctor's pretest instructions are a little different, but they all involve starting with some sort of clear-liquid diet and low-carb eating, because they want to make sure your cells are stimulated in a specific way during the test itself. You will most likely also be asked to refrain from strenuous exercise the day before the test. (Oh damn!) Next is the chalky drink, and then there's an injection of sugar containing radioactive FDG—fluorodeoxyglucose. The injection is through a line they start in your arm. Just a needle prick, not a huge event. The doctors are checking to see how the cells metabolize the sugar in the injection. During the scan the cells are active, and the activity shows up as bright lights on the images. The radiologist is looking for cells that appear abnormally bright. A PET scan may be ordered to look for signs of cancer that were not detected on an MRI or a mammogram.

My favorite part? After they've completed all the

prep, they leave you alone and tell you to relax. This time they really mean "Relax." A darkened room, no reading, no TV. Just you and your thoughts. My test center has a light-up photo of a beach on the wall. The tech turns it on as he leaves, and the water looks like it's moving. All of a sudden, amid the crashing waves, you hear the sound of seagulls calling. I kid you not. The worst part is that the first time I was there, I couldn't figure out how to turn it off. Not exactly soothing. It doesn't work anymore. *Such* a shame (I swear I didn't do it)!

Next stop, the PET room itself. It looks just like the MRI room. Once you're all positioned, and they leave the room and slide you in, you'll hear a recorded voice that tells you when to breathe and when to hold it. "Breathe in. Hold . . ." An hour or so later, "Breathe out." Okay, it's not really an hour. I have no idea how long you actually hold your breath, but they tell you to do the best you can. I decided to turn it into a game. The first time I didn't make it all the way, but after a while I got into the groove. The trick is not to pass out. Then it's time for the pee-in-your-pants sensation. Yup, they'll tell you that when they send the liquid through your arm you may feel a warming sensation through your nether regions. It's a peculiar feeling, and maybe just a little bit funny. But other than that, the test is pretty much a nonevent in terms of its physical toll on you. Wondering about the results takes a whole other toll. This is most likely the first of many PET/CT scans you will have in your life. Post-treatment, these are the follow-up scans they perform regularly to see if the cancer has returned.

TOP 5 TIPS FOR PET/CT SCANS

∽

1. Bring a Xanax (or equivalent antianxiety drug) with you, and take it with the "milk" if you're claustrophobic or anxious.

2. Pee before you start the test, but drink lots and lots of water after. I learned this trick when I had dry mouth for days after my first PET.

3. If you have a PowerPort (everything you ever wanted to know about PowerPorts starts on page 64), ask them to use it for the injections. You may have to have it accessed first by a chemo nurse, but I'm a believer in using that thing every single chance I get.

4. Make sure you've asked a friend or family member to drive you home when it's over. There's nothing truly

---

horrible about this test, and there's no chance of getting results on the spot, but it still takes a lot out of you. Some doctors suggest you stay away from people because you're radioactive, but this never made any sense to me. You're in a cancer center surrounded by people when you have the test to begin with. I guess it couldn't hurt to stay away from other cancer patients or pregnant women for about six hours if possible.

5. There are always snacks available for people who've just had these tests—usually a granola bar or something. Go for it. Eat them. You deserve it. Take one for the car.

BONE SCAN

A bone scan, also called bone scintigraphy, is an imaging test used to determine whether breast cancer has traveled to the bones. Your doctor may order one at initial diagnosis, to make sure your bones are healthy. He or she may also want to create baseline images that can be used for comparison at a later date after treatment. Additionally, a bone scan may be ordered if you have bone and joint pain or a blood test suggests the possibility that the breast cancer has traveled to the bone. In other words, lots of reasons. Always feel free to ask your doctor why this, and any other scan, was or was not ordered.

This one is easy, even for me, and I'm claustrophobic. First they inject a radioactive material into your vein or through your port. They show up with the stuff in this strange metal cylinder, like a mininuke, and then draw it up through a needle. Totally sci-fi. Then you wait an hour for the material to circulate. You don't feel different, and you don't start to glow. After an hour you lie down, and they slide you in and out of yet another tube-like machine. There's no pain, nothing disgusting to drink. It's just dull. The only side effect may be a metallic taste that some people get when they inject the material. Yup, I had that too.

TOP 5 TIPS FOR A BONE SCAN

1. Bring a Tic Tac or hard candy to suck on when they do the injection. It keeps the metallic taste away.

2. Bring a buddy, a book, or your own magazine. You really do have to sit around for at least an hour

---

between the injection and the test. And the waiting room will most likely be filled with old magazines with "what's hot" lists from the year before.

3. Practice relaxation breathing while you're doing the test. There's nothing else to do, and it gives you something to focus on.

4. Don't be polite. If you hate country music, ask them to change the station! Believe me, once you're stuck in there you'll be sorry if you hate "Achy Breaky Heart" and you're listening to it for the third time.

5. Again, pee right before you go in for the test. You're going to thank me for this.

Usually the people who administer these tests are incredibly nice. They ask if you need a blanket or a pillow or anything else. If you can think of something that will make you more comfortable, let them know. If you don't like the technician, ask to see someone else. Seriously. This is not the time to be accommodating.

3

Results

So of course you're hoping it's just the one thing. Just the tumor (or the tumors, in my case). You're praying that no lymph nodes are involved, that it hasn't spread. It's pretty much all you can think about during the tests. My brother is a radiologist, and he says the thing about these tests is that sometimes they can answer questions, and sometimes they create more questions. Lots of things show up on bone scans and PET scans that are not cancer, and sometimes you never find out what those things are. They're anomalies in your body, and they might be perfectly normal, but now you have to worry about them. The doctors see three "somethings" on one scan that they can't explain, so you have a different scan and it eliminates two of the spots. But there's a third, and they don't know what it is, but it doesn't look like cancer. This is exactly what happened to me. My results answered some questions

and raised a few more. What was the third spot? Nobody knew. My oncologist said, "We've taken that
road as far as we can; now we have to turn to what we
do know. This is medicine. You have to accept some
question marks." They don't know everything. It's
really hard to live with, but true.

At this point you'll want to know what stage of
cancer you're in, but if you're having surgery, the doctors won't give you a stage until afterward. They will
talk to you about it, though, and the stages are both
more complicated and less meaningful than I thought.
What your doctor says to you about your cancer is
more important than the stage number.

What you need to know right away is that *all* stages
are treatable. Some stages come with surgery, chemotherapy, and radiation, some with only one or two of
them. But *every* stage is treatable—even stage 4.

The literature now refers to breast cancer as a
chronic disease. Something you can live with for a
long time. This is true. I met lots of people in waiting
rooms who'd been diagnosed ten, fifteen years before.
I found this both encouraging and scary. I was happy
to know I wasn't going to die right away, but I really
couldn't imagine going through treatment for fifteen
years. I guess you do what you have to do.

I do take offense, however, when it's referred to as a chronic disease like diabetes or something similar. Cancer is not like any other disease. It includes, among other things, a huge "dread" factor that most other chronic diseases don't have, and the treatments are not like those for diabetes at all. But you can live with it—many, many people *are* living with it—and there are new trials and drugs literally all the time.

TELLING YOUR FAMILY AND FRIENDS

At the time my husband and I went to see one of the breast surgeons for a consultation, we still hadn't told our kids. I'd known for about ten days and had had a week of tests, but since the surgery hadn't been scheduled, we still hadn't said anything. The surgeon told us we had to tell them. Right away. He said that kids are sensitive, and they'd probably already figured out that something was up. We talked to a social worker, read the pamphlets about how to tell teenagers, and found out we agreed with the consensus. Here it is: Be honest, but put it in a positive light. Mom has been diagnosed with breast cancer, but we're treating it right away. We're lining up a great team of doctors, and although it's scary, this is a treatable disease, and we're doing everything we can to make sure she's going to be okay. And we're going to tell you everything as we go along.

We followed the professional advice we received. We were honest and only offered as much detail as each child requested. Obviously everyone's kids will take the news differently. The social worker said that most will ask a few questions, then pretty much ask what's for dinner. This turned out to be true. My kids reacted according to their personalities. One only wanted the worst-case scenario: "Are you going to die?" The other wanted much more information. One moved on from the news quicker than the other. My daughter, Marisa, jokingly offers the following advice for what to do when you sit your kids down:

Step 1—Here's a cookie.
Step 2—I have cancer, but I'm going to be okay.
Step 3—Here's some money.

Since we had teenagers, we also told them not to search the Internet randomly because there's so much false information. Also, there'd be plenty of information out there that wouldn't apply to me. My son, Jeremy, would occasionally ignore my advice not to research things online, and then get upset by what he found. My daughter only cared about what was actually happening to me, not the statistics. My oncologist recommended that we tell them about www.breastcancer.org if they asked. It has the most up-to-date and scientifically sound information. That's what we did.

Telling the rest of my family was the worst part. There's never a good time to tell someone who loves you that you have cancer. My big worry was that my mother would want to move into my house. That's exactly what she wanted to do. We had to find a balance between her need to take care of me, my need still to be a grown-up, and my husband's need for some privacy. It turns out you have a lot of responsibility when you have cancer. How you present yourself and your disease to your family, friends, and coworkers is often complicated. Of course I wanted to be like the women in those TV miniseries who are fighters and deal with all the treatment and surgery with humor and grace. *Hah!* That's fiction. You know how you tell your kids that the monsters in the movies aren't real? Guess what? The perfect cancer patient in the movie isn't real either. The producers don't show her awake at four a.m., unable to sleep because of pain and side effects and worry. They don't show her yelling at the kids because of steroid rage. So don't set yourself or your family up. Be honest; don't oversell.

This book actually started as a blog on www.car ingbridge.org as a way for me to let everyone outside my immediate circle know how I was doing. I did it partly as a way to cut down on having to tell the story a million times. Or receiving a hundred phone calls a day that started with, "Hi, just checking in to see how you are." I realized very quickly into my deep dive down the rabbit hole that I couldn't handle that.

When you tell people, they'll all respond differently. Some will tell you you'll be fine because you're young and strong. Or old and strong. Or just you. Some will burst into tears. Some will be stoic and offer to do anything they can for you. Some will immediately start talking about people they've known who've had cancer. Some will want to tell you horror stories. And then the advice starts. Some people just *have* to offer advice. A flood of advice. And all of it conflicting. About what you should or shouldn't eat or which doctor to see. About whether or not you should exercise. About how to keep your spirits up (you will hear the words "fighting spirit" way too many times). They cannot help themselves.

If you're like me, you'll find some of it thoughtful

and well intentioned but frustrating and confusing. And you'll want to turn off the spigot. My surgeon's nurse gave me the best advice of all. She told me just to say, "Thank you, but everyone's experience is different, and I'm not comfortable talking about it." For those who want to give you a medical consult, just say, "I'm very comfortable with my doctors, and I'm taking medical advice only from them, but thank you anyway."

Not long after I was in treatment, a woman I had known casually for years and who I knew had been fighting her own battle for all that time wrote me an e-mail that ended with "Welcome to my club." I wrote back, "Your club *sucks*."

SHARING THE NEWS

∞

1. Tell your kids and immediate family right away. Be clear and concise. Keep the script simple. Plan what you're going to say, rehearse it with yourself or someone you trust, and stick to it.

2. Sign up for www.caringbridge.org or one of the other Web sites offered by your local cancer center

---

to use as a clearinghouse for information. Even if you yourself don't use it to write, someone in your immediate circle can do it to keep everyone up-to-date. You can even include photos. I posted ones of me in all my different wigs.

3. Make sure everyone knows your policy on advice. Medical advice should come from your medical team *only*. No exceptions. My brother's a radiologist, and even though he counts as a doctor, I wanted his advice to come through my own oncologist so I had him call my doctor first. Doctors only.

4. Do not answer the phone if you don't want to. It's not your responsibility to listen to everyone's reactions when they find out. Let someone else give you the message: "Dina called; she sends her love." You don't need to listen to twenty minutes of . . . whatever. People say so many things—from the inspirational to the insufferable. Pick and choose carefully.

5. Don't pretend to be something you're not. You're shocked. You're sad and shaken and scared and lots of other *s* words. You will be lots of other letters as well. You don't have to make believe you're okay with breast cancer. Of course you're going to

fight, blah, blah, blah. You got this book, didn't you?
Embrace the fact that your life may stink right now
and you don't have to pretend otherwise.

CHOOSING A SURGEON

The most important thing about choosing the right
surgeon is knowing his or her level of experience in
breast surgery. If possible, choose someone who only
does breast surgery. Breast surgery, like all surgeries,
is part science, part art. Some of what's done in the
operating room is, simply, the surgeon's call, based on
how much what he sees in you corresponds to what he
knows. You'll want someone who has seen almost everything there is to see, done almost everything there
is to do. Make sure you know your surgeon's point
of view as well. Yes, surgeons have a point of view.
Is she known for breast conservation or for being ag-
gressive? Be sure you know where the surgeon's coming from so you can determine if that view meshes
with your own. If possible, get a second opinion from
someone with a different frame of reference so you
can make the choice that feels right to you.

When they remove the tumor, it's all about the
margins, the buffer zone of healthy tissue they take

out with the tumor to make sure they've got it all. You need someone who can not only recognize where the margins of the tumor are, but who is skilled and practiced enough to know how to take out just the right amount of tissue, no more, no less. In addition, some types of surgery require "sentinel node biopsies," where the surgeon takes out specific lymph nodes—sentinels are a kind of early-warning system—to perform an on-the-spot test for signs of cancer. Your surgeon needs to be able to determine the right sentinel nodes in your case. With all this going on, you can see why experience is paramount.

Finally, make sure the pathology lab in your surgeon's hospital has a great reputation. These are the people who will be doing the tests that determine the type of tumor you have, as well as whether there is node involvement. If they don't have a great rep, you have two choices: (1) choose another surgeon; (2) have the lab results sent out for a second opinion.

Do your homework. Find out who the head of breast surgery is, and meet with him or her. Ask everyone who the best surgeons are, and meet with them. I asked the radiologist who did my MRI, my oncologist, my friends. Then we met the people they recommended and chose the one we were most comfortable with. This is one time in your life when reputation is key.

Keep in mind that there is an advantage to having your oncologist and breast surgeon in the same hospital. Hospitals have tumor boards that meet weekly, and they discuss the cancer cases. If your oncologist and your breast surgeon are affiliated with the same hospital, all your records are under the same roof, and they can easily get in touch with each other if they need to.

At the end of the day you have to feel comfortable with the hospital, the surgeon, and her staff. This does not mean you have to like her. You'll only have a few interactions with your surgeon, so personality is far less important than the results of her work. This isn't *Gray's Anatomy*. This is your life. You just have to feel confident that she knows what she's doing.

I met with two surgeons before I picked one. They both had superior reputations, and they were both obviously highly skilled. One was like a breast surgeon rock star. (Wonder what *those* concert T-shirts would look like?!) He was such a star that he'd left the big hospital, wooed by a smaller place to build its reputation. Good for him, bad for my boob. I didn't like the smaller hospital. I was worried about the quality of his support. The staff in the operating room comes from the hospital, as do the people in intensive care. I wanted the best of both worlds. I chose the surgeon from my oncologist's hospital, the one who told us he was a truffle hunter on weekends. Why he told me this, I don't know, but for some reason it made a difference. In the end it really doesn't matter what they say until they say something that makes you more or less comfortable.

TOP 5 TIPS FOR CHOOSING A SURGEON

1. Being able to talk to a human being, not voice mail, goes a long way toward a positive experience. When you call your surgeon with a question, you want a person on the other end. My surgeon has two nurses on staff to answer patient questions. It was invaluable to know that I could always call and one of them would be there to talk to.

2. You will have about six weeks of aftercare with your surgeon, so you'd better feel comfortable with him or her. That still doesn't mean you have to like him

---

or her. You need to feel confident in the surgeon's education, skills, and knowledge. You should feel heard and treated like a human being. But at the end of the day you don't need to love your surgeon—just his work.

3. If the differences are negligible, or if you don't know how else to choose, pick the surgeon with the hospital where you feel the care is the best.

4. Research the reputation of the pathology lab in the hospital where your surgeon works. Ask other doctors, friends, relatives, and so on to learn what you can. If you hear something you don't like, ask the surgeon about it. The response may give you something to go on.

5. After you do the research and decide, stop fretting. Even if lots of other people talk about some other rock-star surgeon, it doesn't matter. You've done your homework and made the best choice for you.

4

Surgery

ONE LUMP OR TWO?
AND OTHER AGONIZING CHOICES

Your diagnosis may give you some answers, but it can also lead to many more questions. Lumpectomy or mastectomy? Single or double? Reconstruction or prosthesis? Which surgeon? Oncologist? And so on and so on. . . . All of a sudden you're presented with life-altering choices. You will probably find yourself wondering: How am I supposed to make these decisions, and why am I the one being asked?

First of all, there's one overall reason that your doctor will ask you to make some of these choices: There's no compelling medical reason to choose one option over another. *Whaaat?* you may ask. You're telling me modern medicine doesn't have all the answers? It does not. When there's no medical reason to sway your doctor in one direction, the deciding factor turns out to be your own lifestyle choices.

Since my surgery and treatment, I have often revisited the literature and asked for more medical opinions on removing my left (and so far cancer-free) breast. All the specialists keep telling me the same thing: There's no medical reason for removing it, but it's up to you. So here I am, left (pun intended) with one breast and one scar and a drawer full of prostheses. Here's my opinion, for what it's worth: There are huge pros and cons no matter what your choice. Helpful, right?

On the one hand, I enjoy having sensation on the left side of my chest. The anxiety I feel about the cancer returning has nothing to do with that lonely breast over there. I would not feel any more secure about my future if it was removed because once you've seen the great and powerful Oz, you know you're not in Kansas anymore and this is no Technicolor dream you can wake up from. This is real. On the other hand, having one breast is something I'm always managing around. If I'm not wearing a prosthesis, I'm wearing a flowy shirt and scarf for camouflage. I wouldn't say I'm used to it after all this time, but I've learned to manage. Which leads to the next choice you will have to make:

RECONSTRUCTION

This is a big topic. I, unfortunately, was not a candidate for immediate reconstruction because of the radiation

I had to receive. This happens to many women, but as far as I can tell, it's rarely discussed. Everyone just assumes that reconstruction is an option for everyone and that everybody does it. Not true. In 2007, 63 percent of women undergoing mastectomy opted for reconstruction.* That means there's a whopping 37 percent of us walking around with either one boob or none. For some it was a choice. For others there was no choice. Either radiation caused too much tissue damage, or continued medications inhibit healing, or many other reasons. So if you're like me, and reconstruction wasn't on your list of menu choices, don't worry—you are not alone.

If, on the other hand, you have the option of reconstruction—lucky you? Yes, that question mark is there on purpose. You get more choices: (1) autologous reconstruction (using tissue from your own body); (2) implants; (3) stem cells and fat tissue. (I have plenty of fat and fat tissue, if anyone needs my help.) All these options have their risks and benefits, and if you have the option of starting the process during the mastectomy, those choices need to be made quickly.

* *Journal of Clinical Oncology*, February 18, 2013.

If you don't have to have radiation following surgery, my advice is to talk to plastic surgeons about reconstruction *before* your mastectomy. There may be skin-sparing or nipple-sparing procedures that your surgeon should perform if you are having reconstruction soon after a mastectomy. You can have implants or expanders, skin grafts, and many other options, and you should discuss them all with your doctors. It may seem like a daunting task to have these conversations right at the very beginning, but that's the time to do it. Get two or three opinions, talk to your breast surgeon for referrals, friends, and the like. Make sure the plastic surgeons you talk to have specific experience with breast cancer reconstruction. This is not the time to consult with the Beverly Hills doc who specializes in double Ds.

If you're reading this book in the early stages of diagnosis, take a breath here and do the research. Make sure that you're totally comfortable with the plastic surgeon doing your reconstruction, and that he or she is experienced in breast reconstruction, not just breast augmentation surgery. This is not the same thing as a Beverly Hills housewife wanting a pair of new boobs for Christmas. I told my husband I didn't mind having my mastectomy in Seattle, but if I was getting a boob job, I was going to Los Angeles. We even drew pictures of what we thought boob jobs looked like across the country. I wanted grade-A California boobs, but it turns out that's not the best way to pick a surgeon.

Breast reconstruction is a surgical specialty. A lumpectomy or mastectomy creates an entirely different surgical landscape than just regular implants. Number one, you have to be prepared to accept some level of asymmetry. In fact, your breasts are asymmetrical now if they're natural, but you're probably used to them. Once you start focusing on redesigning them, you kind of want them to be perfect. However, reconstruction is an imperfect art. The outside world won't be able to see the imperfections, but you will.

They do *amazing* things with reconstruction these days. Create new nipples, tattoo a new areola, lift, reduce, enlarge. The results can be extremely realistic. All plastic surgeons have before-and-after pictures for you to peruse. Just think—you may be America's Next Topless Model!

TOP 5 TIPS FOR
CHOOSING YOUR SURGERY

∽

1. Research all your surgical and nonsurgical options. Be sure to ask about the timing option for everything.

2. Meet several plastic surgeons and look at all the photos. Make sure you know what you're getting.

3. Ask about nipple options. Will they save yours or tattoo one on? Look at all the photos of the tattoos. Ask about 3-D tattooing—yes, this is a real thing. Your surgeon may know someone who does this.

4. Don't let yourself feel pressured by the timing. It's a big decision, and although it may be an option to start reconstruction during the mastectomy surgery, you may not be ready to make that decision in the midst of fighting for your life. Do what feels best to you.

5. If you have a life partner, this can be a tricky conversation. Both of you need to look at the photos and make peace with your decision. Don't forget, though, no matter what decision you make, a reconstructed breast following a radical mastectomy

has no feeling. Sometimes women who have re-construction using a flap have some small areas of feeling return after a while; for the most part it's for display purposes only.

BEFORE

How can I tell you how to prepare for one of the most dramatic changes of your life? The most annoying thing to me was that all the books, and even the surgeon and some survivors I met, kept telling me that the surgery was the easiest part. You have *got* to be kidding! Yes, I know it's a relatively simple surgery, but it's my breast and you are cutting it off! I agree it's the shortest part of the experience, but it's not necessarily the easiest. You know your hair will grow back after chemo, but your breasts don't grow back. Even if reconstruction is an option for you, things will never be the same. You *will* get used to the new you—but it will take time.

There are so many fears and questions. Simple fear of surgery, for one. Fear of pain and discomfort and scarring, for another. Then there's the whole idea that your body will forever be altered, and you can't help wondering what it will really look like. There's a whole lot of anxiety for you and for anyone who might see you naked. The books all say to discuss it openly. Easier said than done. Still, it's vital to be able to talk about it.

Everybody responds differently and needs different things, but I can tell you what I did. I decided to take some time to myself and try to put it all in perspective. I took two days to focus on what was going to happen to me. I drove to the beach and walked along the shore. I stood in front of the mirror with my hand covering my breast, trying to picture what it would look like. I looked at photos in books and online. I didn't want to be shocked when I saw myself. Look, it's still shocking and dramatic. You can't change that, but you can prepare yourself so you have some buffer against the shock. I tied my hair up in a scarf and tried to envision myself bald. I think it helped me to just take the time to get ready for the onslaught. You don't necessarily need two days, but you might need more than two hours. By yourself, just to come to terms.

DURING

The morning of surgery you and your loved ones are most likely going to be on emotional high alert. Feelings of dread and anxiety plagued me the night before and the morning of my surgery, and right up until they knocked me out in the operating room. Any surgery is a little scary, this one even more so because *this* surgery has that big "cancer" word attached to it. *This* surgery has the added component of determining your next course of treatment. *This* surgery might tell you if the cancer has spread or not. It's not like they're fixing something that's broken. You usually don't go into the hospital feeling perfectly fine, knowing that by the end of the day you'll feel lousy. *This* surgery is scary.

I went to the hospital with my husband and my parents. The kids went to school, and I went to surgery. It was a very peculiar feeling to say good-bye to them like it was a normal school day, and then get in the car and head to the hospital for the beginning of the most dramatic chapter of our lives. I was more than a little nervous. I knew I'd wake up minus a boob and plus a port. I'd tried to find out as much as I could, looking at lots of images online and trying to wrap my head around what was happening, but I had only the vaguest idea what that would look or feel like. Also, we knew that we'd find out about the tumor's characteristics and what stage I was, officially. It's a lot to take in. The nurse who did my prep work was a survivor, which helped. Not only that, but she told me she still had her port in, seven years later. She'd just never bothered to have it removed. I have to say that made me feel a little better about the port. The fact that she wasn't anxious to get it out meant that it couldn't be that bad. Also, at that moment, seven years seemed like a long time—a *very* long time.

In the movies and on TV, they always wheel the patient toward the operating room, and the spouse walks next to the gurney and kisses her just before they whisk her away. Guess what? It doesn't always work like that anymore. I had to walk into the operating room. Right, walk in there and lie down on the table. Apparently this is how it's done in many hospitals. Is there a gurney shortage or something? I guess if you walk yourself into the hospital for surgery, you get to walk yourself into the operating room. Never mind the fact that your legs are shaking and your heart is pounding. I, of course, wanted to be one of those patients whom the nurses and doctors would describe later as brave and funny. I felt the need to banter and make terrible jokes. Not exactly sure why I felt the need to put on a show for the people cutting me open, but I think I wanted them to like me so they'd do an extra-good job.

When you wake up, you shouldn't be in pain

because you'll be jacked up on meds. The procedure is not complicated, and the hospital's view is that most people just—well—deal with it. Not much hospital care for a mastectomy, which is kind of strange to me. I mean, it is essentially an amputation, right? They just removed an exterior part of my body, so I thought of it as a breast amputation. It comes with all the phantom nipple feelings and other weird stuff like an amputation, so that's what it felt like to me. I just kept repeating to myself, "Life first, boob second."

Post-surgery, your chest may be wrapped up a little with a kind of Ace bandage thing. They teach you something about your drain—a plastic contraption that is inserted with tubing into the surgical site to drain off fluid that accumulates under the skin after surgery—and they give you meds to deal with your pain. And then off you go. A little bit lighter than before. Physically, anyway. If you're in a great deal of pain, or need another tutorial on the drain, tell a nurse. Make sure you're confident in your ability to care for yourself at home before you leave.

THE DRAIN

The most important thing to know about this contraption is that it is not as disgusting as you imagine. Really. Having said that, nothing prepared me for the experience of living with an annoying plastic football-shaped device attached to me. At least it's not that big—just a few inches long.

At some point shortly after surgery, a nurse will teach you how to "milk" the drain—more than a little ironic considering you've just lost your milk ducts. The drain starts as plastic tubing that protrudes out of your side (or both sides, if you had a double mastectomy) that's meant to allow the fluid that accumulates during the healing process to drain. Attached to the end of the tubing is a pump that draws out the excess fluid into a receptacle vessel. Mine looked like a little football. The tubing is attached to your skin with a little stitch that will give new meaning to the phrase, "I have a stitch in my side." Inside your body the drain tubing runs from that little incision up under your arm, then loops back and into your chest area behind where your breast used to be.

You may experience some postsurgical pain under your arm and under the surgery site; it may be caused by this tubing. Nobody warned me about that. I had to figure it out for myself. I had pain in my armpit and couldn't understand why for quite a while. The thing about the tubing in you is that it moves, so you will occasionally get a sharp pain or tugging feeling, and you just have to try to move around until it changes again. It's not pleasant.

A lot of women are worried about doing the milking of the drain and think it's disgusting. Quite a few I spoke to had their husbands do it. I didn't think it was that big a deal. If you've changed diapers, you've done far worse. It's just fluid with some blood in it. You don't touch it; you just see it.

All you do is kind of squeeze the tubing from the top into the drain, like flattening the kinks out of a rope or hose. That's it. You're just pinching your fingers together and running them down the length of the little hose—okay, so it's a little gross—and then you measure the fluid, and keep a log. My surgeon finally told me I didn't have to be perfectly exact, just do the best I could. I was sure that every drop mattered in the measurement, but it doesn't. Just picture me in the bathroom with the little measuring thing they give you, trying to decide if I should put it on the counter and lean over or bring it up to eye level. I mean, is it measuring for baking or just stir-fry? Because they're different. The most important thing is that you do it at about the same time every day and that you don't let the drain back up or the football get too full, because that can cause infection.

When you milk the drain and measure (roughly) the contents, you're doing it to see when your body stops creating the fluid that fills the incision site. When the flow slows down enough, the surgeon will remove the drain. This is painless. Yay, painless! I cheer for anything that doesn't hurt.

Don't worry about how long it takes for the surgeon to decide to remove it. My drain was in forever! I felt like a kangaroo carrying its young in a pouch. I hated talking to women who said, "Oh, the drain, that was nothing. I had mine out in a few days." Mine stayed in for four weeks! And then we finally took it out, and I still had to go in for aspirations. This is where they stick a needle in the pillow of fluid that has now formed under your arm, and they drain it. The great news is that you feel *nothing*. It does not hurt at all. The other news: The sound of the liquid draining into the metal pan can be gross. Plus, don't look. That *is* gross.

It took me at least a week to figure out that I should sit on the side of the car where the seat belt crossed my healthy side. I had surgery on my right side, which meant I had to sit in the backseat behind the driver until I had healed. *Duhhh*. Sit on the side of the car where the seat belt doesn't dig into your surgical site.

AFTER

Pain. Right after the surgery in the hospital, when you've got all your pain meds on board, it doesn't hurt that much. Then you get home and those meds start to wear off, and it hurts. Nobody has the same response to pain as you do, but it hurts. Your body has just been traumatized. Take the medication religiously as prescribed, and try not to overdo it physically. Seriously, you just had surgery. What did you expect?

Ready for some good news? At least for me it really didn't hurt as much as I thought it would, because (something I'd forgotten) the skin covering the area of my surgery went numb. The surgeon warned me this would happen. To do a mastectomy he has to cut nerves, and they don't come back. So the skin itself is numb across that whole area. And if you had lymph nodes removed—which means he had to expand his work to the armpit—you're numb under your arm as well. For me it's going to stay that way permanently. I wish I could tell you that there's no pain at all, but that'd be a huge, ugly lie. But there's less than I imagined. So take this as a little blessing. In fact, you need to start counting your little blessings, and this is as good a place to start as any.

Even more important, this is when you hear about

everything the doctor learned during the surgery. You still have to wait for the results of some tests. But certain things are now known. You want to hear your surgeon say the magic words "clean margins." That's his way of telling you he thinks he got the whole tumor, with a little room to spare. Surgeons tend to be very proud of their work and their margins. They like to brag about all the stuff they did to you and how well they did it. If the guy's saving my life, I'm open to a little bragging, but it's still my body that's been assaulted, no matter how well he thinks it came out. And of course you're waiting to hear what they found in your lymph nodes, whether they think the cancer has spread, what stage you are, and what kind of cancer it is. No way around the freakiness of that, I'm afraid.

What the *hell* does it look like, anyway? A big slash across your chest. And the whole area is just *sooo* flat. It's so flat that it looks concave. It's not, but your experience of what it looks like may be that it's almost receded. It's just that you're used to having something protruding and, now, when your arm is up, you can actually see the curve of your back. So it really is flatter than your mind assumes it will be before you actually see it.

I'm going to tell you to look at yourself as soon as you can. It's not going to get easier until you get used to it. Your surgeon is going to make it as aesthetically pleasing as possible, and you can't hide from your own body, so you might as well start now. It's not ugly or disgusting. You're just going to see a red slash and some stitches and maybe a little bruising.

The tiny area where they inserted the drain and stitched it in place becomes a scar. I never really thought about it, and it doesn't matter because it's so small, but it's real, and nobody told me about it. Also, some people (and of course this was me) get a kind of depression (no, not a mood swing—I'll talk plenty about those later—but an actual physical dent) a few inches below the armpit from the removal of lymph nodes and breast tissue. It's totally fine. You'd only see it if I'm naked and raise my arm above my head and point it out to you (which I very rarely do).

Every surgeon sends his patients home with a slightly different dressing. Mine was almost nothing, just a tiny flap of gauze and some sterile tape. My surgeon believes in air-drying the surgical site. And, yes, the thing oozes. Not a lot, just a little.

The reality is that it's just skin and scabbing and healing and dealing with the drain. Don't be afraid of what you see. Nothing about the incision site has anything to do with cancer, so don't be surprised when your surgeon talks about the margins and then moves on. For him the rest is all about the business of healing: drainage and scarring and scabbing.

A blood blister can form in the scar. This happened to me. One of the spots in the incision area just didn't drain and dry the same way as the rest did, and a little pocket formed. It was almost black but eventually it leaked, then healed. Now you can't even tell.

The other thing you will learn about in your surgeon's office is the importance of doing stretching exercises. You have to get mobility back in your arm, and the only way to do it is to stretch. I want to know why reaching for the cookie jar doesn't aid healing, but apparently you have to "walk" your fingers up a wall a few times a day. (Maybe if you put the cookie jar on a shelf on the wall that would work?) Seriously, though, if you don't stretch, you can heal so tightly that you lose some mobility around your arm. I figured I'd lost enough already since I was minus a breast, so I did the exercises. I also looked into the physical therapy options at my cancer center and checked with my insurance to see what they would cover.

GETTING DRESSED

How to fake it in the beginning: Get a postsurgical camisole. It's a white fabric tank top with a pocket on either side, into which you insert a "puff" (for a while, this is your new boob). The puff—yes, that's what they call it—is a round cotton pocket filled with stuffing that Velcros into the camisole. It also has a pouch in the front where you put your drain. So now you have a pouch and a puff. Sounds like a marsupial of some kind, but no, it's you. Your surgeon's staff should be able to tell you where you can find them locally. Sometimes there's a store right in the hospital, and even your local Nordstrom's has supplies. Right, Nordy's. Get two so you can have a clean one every day. It's doable. Just keep in mind that your remaining breast is swinging free on the other side. You cannot wear a bra for quite a while because you can't wear anything tight around the incision site.

POSTSURGICAL FOLLOW-UP

The most annoying and uncomfortable part of the follow-up is that your surgeon is tapping and poking you, and although the skin is numb, there is a really bizarre kind of toothache-feeling beneath the skin. So it doesn't exactly hurt, but it does not feel good. Oh no it doesn't! The surgeon also may need to trim the scab that forms on the incision. I discovered on my own that if you sterilize a pair of toenail or nail clippers with rubbing alcohol (you know, the ninety-nine-cent kind you get at the drugstore), they work way better than the surgical scissors the doctors use, and it hurts a lot less. You just clip off the part of the scab that's sticking up too far—you'll know what I mean when it happens to you—and it doesn't tug or pull or hurt at all. My surgeon will kill me for telling you to do that, but I stand by it.

Keep doing the exercises. There's going to be a day when you get up and realize you are starting to feel like you can do laundry and reach for things on the highest shelf. *Don't* do it until weeks after surgery. Keep protecting that side. Another ongoing theme: Think of the short run vs. long run and decide in favor of the long run. Yes, the short run sucks, but you can get through it.

TOP 5 TIPS FOR
BEFORE AND AFTER A MASTECTOMY

∽

1. Get a washable—or very light—fanny pack, or a waterproof cell phone case with a long strap for the shower. When you shower with the drain in, you

have to put it somewhere. If it's not supported, it hangs and drags on you, and that does not feel good. My surgeon gave me a little fabric pouch with a long ribbon strap to hang around my shoulder in the shower. Huge help.

2. The tendons and muscles that connect your arm to your pectoral muscles can form a kind of ribbon of scar tissue. Some doctors refer to this as "cording." It's what you're stretching when you do your exercises. It can get tight overnight or in an hour. Or be fine for a week and then get tight, and you can actually see it. You just have to keep moving it and stretching, and it will ease up again, but the tightness that develops is what the term "frozen" refers to in the literature.

3. After the incision is really starting to heal, get some A+D ointment and apply it to the scab and scar. It will help soften the scar and help the skin to heal.

4. You will get weird pains in your arm and hand from out of nowhere as the nerves start to grow back. The best description I heard came from my surgeon, who told me (only after I asked) that his patients said there are small pains and big pains, shooting pains,

sticking pains, tingling pains, and aching pains. They come and go and they're all pains, but they're normal, and most are quick to pass.

5. Don't overdo it. Surgery is just the beginning of your journey. Do your best to recover from this as well as you can, because the next phase is longer and has more side effects than the surgery itself. Most likely you won't be allowed to start chemotherapy until after you're pretty well healed anyway. Nobody wants complications or infections to interfere with chemo or healing.

BRA SHOPPING

Should you choose to forgo reconstruction, or like me, have that decision made for you, you will now have the joy of prosthesis fitting. This section is mainly for those of you who, like me, had a single mastectomy and have to deal with the lopsidedness. After you get past the drain-plus-cotton-puff stage, you still have to get dressed every day. If you have to wait to wear a bra until after radiation, you may actually become used to swinging in the breeze and dressing to hide the discrepancy. However, there comes a point in every single-boob girl's life where she has to go out and get the correct breast prosthesis and find the bras that suit it.

I thought bra companies would make several categories of bras to be worn with prostheses. After all, there are a lot of us single (breasted) girls, right? There'd be the sexy, Victoria's Secret version, the old-fashioned kind, and the medical-supply-store version. Nope. It turns out there's only one, and it's pretty much a marriage between the old-fashioned and the medical-supply kind. Of course Nordstrom's is happy to come to your rescue. Each store has a consultant in the lingerie department trained to fit you and your flatness. And Nordy's will submit the paperwork for your insurance as well. Oh, yes, it's important to know that you need a prescription for a fake boob. Right there on the prescription pad above your surgeon's messy signature scrawl, it will say "One Fake Boob." (I'm assuming it actually said "Breast Prosthesis," but I can't be sure—surgeon's handwriting.)

There are other places where this can be done for you. Your local cancer center probably has a list, but I checked out a couple in my neck of the woods and then ran as fast as I could to Nordy's. First of all, I don't understand why the women who work at the stores specializing in prosthesis and mastectomy bras have to have huge, pendulous breasts. I visited a few, and it's like a conspiracy. It seemed like those saleswomen, who were trying to be so kind, were actually mocking me with their breasts. This is not to say you can't have a pleasant experience wherever you go. Most likely you will encounter sympathetic women who want to help you. It's just that the whole experience is kind of traumatic by its very nature, so I preferred Nordstrom's, where I could at least be in a setting with a fluffy robe and a velvet chair to rest in.

It was not what I expected. I somehow thought that you buy the prosthesis and then you can wear whatever bra you want. They actually have prostheses that stick to your skin with silicone dots so you don't need a pocket sewn into your bra to hold it in. I figured my appointment would be about a one-hour deal. *Sooo* wrong!

First you have to find the right prosthesis, and there are different brands with different shapes and weights. You have to pick the one that's closest to your natural shape. Notice I say "closest," because nothing will match you exactly. Then you start trying on bras, because it turns out that not all bras fit your real breast *and* the fake one. Most of the ones that fit both are hideously ugly. I am seriously thinking of starting a line of bras for breast cancer survivors that won't make you look like a 1950s Playtex commercial.

You can have a pocket sewn into some bras that will fit a nonstick prosthesis, but you cannot wear those with a stick-on one because the pocket gets in the way. Your stick-on prosthesis should come with a liner that you can use to allow it to go in a bra pocket, but keep in mind that these prostheses are heavy. Also, you cannot wear the silicone stick-on right after surgery or radiation because it can be irritating to the skin. No matter how lovely the person attending you during this shopping expedition, it is still exhausting and depressing. Just another reminder that nothing is simple (or even pretty) during breast cancer.

I wasn't sure what a prosthesis would actually look like. It's not like I had ever seen one before. Like you, I had never even thought about one before. I didn't even know there was such a thing. If I had imagined one, my fantasy prosthesis would probably have been skin-colored—including an anatomically correct-looking nipple. I certainly wouldn't have pictured the triangular pink-toned molded silicone blob, with a tiny raised dot for a nipple, that actually appeared in my dressing room. There's nothing lifelike about the breast form (that's the official terminology) when it's sitting in the box, but once you wear it in your bra under clothes, it can be remarkable.

In all seriousness it makes a huge (or in my case, B-cup) difference to have something other than a fiberfill puff in your bra. However, be forewarned—a silicone prosthesis in a pocket sewn into a bra is heavy. Even the lightweight ones have some heft to them. It's like carrying around a water balloon all day. By the end of the day when I would take off the wig and the boob, there was a real *aaahhh* feeling. Like taking off your high heels after—wait, no, it's nothing like that at all. It's like taking the elastic out of your ponytail after a long—wait, no, not that, either. It's like unbuttoning your pants after a big meal and—wait, no. Not that, either. It's like none of those things. It's a heavy, fake boob in a pocket in my bra, for crying out loud! But you get the idea. There's a sense of physical relief at the end of the day when all the accoutrements that make you look normal are removed.

Can you feel the difference? *You* can, but nobody

else will. Believe me, I've done the research. I made my husband hug me from all different vantage points, and he swore he couldn't tell. That moment when someone approaches you with outstretched arms may now trigger some apprehension, but I can promise you other people will not feel the prosthesis when they hug you. Of course *you'll* notice, because it pushes against your chest wall, and that sensation is very different from your natural breast. I still find hugging to be slightly awkward, but the pros definitely outweigh the cons!

LYMPH NODES AND YOUR ARM

If you had your lymph nodes taken out like I did, you are in a whole other world of pain and tightness and fear. Fear of what the pathology will reveal and also fear of lymphedema.

I was terrified of lymphedema, the chronic swelling of the arm that can occur after some or all of the lymph nodes are removed. The simple explanation is that the lymphatic fluid has to find new pathways, and sometimes it doesn't. When this happens, the fluid builds up and your arm swells. It's a chronic problem. Once you have it, it won't go away, so the idea is to try to prevent it. However, like cancer, you can do all the right things and still get it. The truth is that a certain percentage of people develop lymphedema, and all you can do is try your best not to be one of them. You should do everything you can to protect yourself. Forever. Sorry, but it's true. Lymphedema can develop at any time. Even years later.

There are exercises and self-massages, all of which you should try. The first person who tried to teach me about all this stuff was a consultant in my surgeon's office. She was well meaning and went into excruciating detail about the lymphatic system. I didn't understand a word she said. Well, that's not exactly true. I understood everything she said, just not why she was saying it. I could have gone to medical school and still not been able to follow it. I later found out that this is a common occurrence. I don't know what it is about the lymphatic system that attracts some of the most humorless and obscure people, but do not be alarmed if you run into one. Keep looking; there's probably another person nearby who can translate for you.

The pamphlet I was given at the hospital was kind of scary, warning me of all sorts of horrible consequences of lymphedema. But the fact is you shouldn't take it lightly, and you can do a few things to help prevent it—*and you should do them all*!

TOP 5 TIPS FOR
PREVENTING LYMPHEDEMA

∞

1. Do not use the arm on the surgical side more than you should. Follow your doctor's orders right from the beginning about limited activity for that arm. Do the arm circles and stretches. It only takes a minute and makes a *huge* difference.

2. Get a compression sleeve for your arm and hand. Your doctor needs to prescribe it, and, for some reason, not all of them do. Ask for it. Insist if you must. The one for your hand is called a gauntlet. The sleeve is like a really tight stocking you wear on your arm. Wear both the sleeve and the gauntlet whenever you do any repetitive activity or exercise. One woman told me I should wear them when I whip cream. Okay, first of all I wonder—do I look like someone who whips cream? What's wrong with the kind that comes out of the can? The fact is, a few months later I was having a dinner party, and, sure enough, there I was with whisk in hand. Of course I was whipping egg whites, but still . . . All of a sudden I panicked—no gauntlet, and I'd been whipping

for three minutes already! I ran to put it on. My arm was fine. The chocolate mousse was not.

3. Learn to protect that hand and arm now, because you will need to protect them for the rest of your life. No blood-draws, blood pressure cuffs, finger sticks, bad cuticles, cheap manicures, tattoos, old razors under the arm, thin pot holders, none of that. You just have to start practicing protection. Try to learn some simple exercises for lymphatic massage. The basic idea is that you want to keep the flow of everything headed back to where there's more room—that is, toward your chest and torso. There are often lymphedema centers around town that can help you as well. Check with your doctor.

4. Use the electric razor you bought to shave your head to shave under your arm. Mine is a pink wet-dry that I got at Target. I've used it for multiple places. Not great for legs, though.

5. Look into the physical therapy that's available at your hospital (mine was covered by insurance for the first several visits, which is all you really need). The exercises you'll learn are very simple. And you won't get a giant arm from physical therapy. It will teach you how to exercise your arm correctly.

THE PORT (OR PORT-A-CATH)

If you're going to have chemotherapy, someone should ask you to consider having a port. The port is a round, dome-like device implanted somewhere near your collarbone. It gives the nurses a reliable place to stick all their needles. It's attached to a catheter that runs under your skin and into one of your veins, providing more direct and easier access to your circulatory system than the veins in your arm. It is a much better and less painful way to receive chemotherapy and give blood for tests. It looks like a round bump under your skin about the size of a nickel. It's definitely kind of a creepy Frankenstein thing, but totally worth it. Ports can be placed on either side of the body in the upper chest, just below the collarbone. The surgeon will decide on which side to place the port based on your anatomy, previous surgery, and location of cancer. This is done during a surgical procedure. Ask your surgeon if you can have it implanted during your mastectomy so you don't have to have an additional procedure. It's barely noticeable. I'd had mine for more than a year before my son pointed at it when I was wearing a T-shirt and said, "Mom, what *is* that thing?" I said, "That's my port." He responded,

"It looks like some alien implanted it." Yup, but for more than a year he hadn't even noticed I'd been abducted by aliens.

Normally it doesn't hurt to have a port, but occasionally it does. The skin over the port itself can be sensitive, especially after a blood draw or chemo; and once in a while you might feel some pain at the point where the catheter runs under your skin near your neck. It goes away quickly, but I did occasionally become aware of discomfort there. Also, avoid direct impact on the port. Touching it is just plain weird because it's definitely a foreign body, but you get used to it.

The doctors sent me home with a little booklet and packet about my port, but didn't tell me much else. It turns out that each one has a number that lets the hospital staff know whether it's a PowerPort or not (which determines the kinds of things they can use it for), and you need to have that information with you. There's a little ID card in the packet that you should put in your wallet and carry around. I wish they'd mentioned that to me in the beginning, because the first time I went to have it accessed, the nurse asked me if it was a Power-Port and where my ID card was. Yes, I got carded at chemo. Now it's in my wallet at all times.

ACCESSING THE PORT/LAB WORK

In my hospital, and in many others, the oncology wing is its own universe. There's a special lab for cancer patients, and it uses the same waiting room as the oncologists. This is where you look around the room at the women wearing wigs and hats and looking well and not so well. You begin to see the same people week after week as you go through your process. It is here that things are both depressing and encouraging. There are always stories to be heard about long illnesses and ongoing treatments. Be careful where you sit. This is the place where you hear the good and the bad and realize you are one of the ugly. I still hate walking into that waiting room to visit my oncologist. It's hard to believe I belong there.

When you go to the lab for tests and need your port accessed, the technician will probably ask you if you want a numbing shot first. Before I knew better, I said, "Absolutely." I mean, who wouldn't want a numbing shot, right? Sign me up! What else can I numb? The thing is, the shot itself was more painful than accessing the port without it. It's two needle sticks instead of one. And the lidocaine itself stings like crazy when it's pushed in with a needle. I think they have to offer it, but I'm a pain wimp and even I said no the second time around. When I hear someone say yes, I always want to lean over and say, "Just say no," but I assume this would be considered bad manners. There is a lidocaine cream your doctor can prescribe called EMLA. You apply it to the port about ninety minutes before your appointment, and voilà, numb! Spread the joy.

To access your port, the technician takes a needle attached to a bit of plastic tubing, punctures the port, and then checks for blood return. To do this she attaches a syringe to the tubing, squeezes in some saline solution, then pulls the plunger back to see if blood enters the syringe (a good thing). Then she takes a few vials of blood for tests and sends you on your way. If you're having other work done, she leaves the tubing in and tapes it to your chest. Then, for the rest of the day, all anyone has to do is attach the lines to the tubing that's already there. When you're done, they just pull the needle out. It's kind of weird because it reminds me of pulling a plunger out. It doesn't hurt, it just makes a clicking sound, and there isn't really a tugging sensation, but it feels like there should be. That part you barely feel at all.

PORT WHINES
(SORRY—MY HUSBAND'S PUN)

Sometimes the darn thing just won't work. The port can get some kind of enzyme buildup on the inside, or get too close to the wall of the vein or something, and when they pull back on the plunger, nothing happens. No blood appears, which means they haven't achieved access. I have a theory that it happens more often when I'm dehydrated, but sometimes it just happens. Then the fun starts. The nurse will practically have you doing calisthenics, hands up, down, lie on this side, roll over, stand up, sit down. *Fight! Fight! Fight!* If nothing else works, she can inject you with an enzyme that removes the buildup, and after about thirty to forty-five minutes, she tries again and you'll probably be good to go. In the meantime there's a lot of suction and pressure on that port, so don't be surprised if you're a little sore after one of these episodes. It's kind of upsetting, only because whenever something varies from the norm, it's unsettling. But it's not a big deal; just go with it.

TOP 5 TIPS FOR DEALING
WITH A PORT

∞

1. Don't be afraid to be high maintenance in the lab. Little things can make a huge difference in making you more comfortable during a very uncomfortable experience. Most of the time the nurses are wonderful and happy to be accommodating. If you come across one who isn't, ask politely for someone else. In some labs you can request a certain nurse each time. Tell the nurse beforehand if you have very sensitive skin. There are hypoallergenic bandages and tapes they can use if you mention it. Also, the Betadine scrubbing pad they often use can irritate your skin, so I just ask them not to use the scrubby thing. Another tip: If they don't wait until the skin protectant dries before putting on a bandage, it can be really itchy, so make sure the nurse waits for it to dry. All adhesives can be irritating if they're put on the skin too quickly. Don't let the nurse just peel off the backing and slap it on you; make sure the air gets to it for a few seconds first.

2. Before you go to have your port accessed for anything, have your doctor give you a prescription for EMLA. It's a numbing cream, and it's fantastic. Make sure you slather a thick layer on your port about an hour and a half before your procedure. Ask the pharmacy if they have any Tegaderm patches to put over the area while the cream is on (I would often ask the nurses during chemo if I could grab an extra one for next time because they usually have a box of them). If you can't get any, just take a piece of plastic wrap and some surgical tape and cover the area. You want to leave a big blob of white cream over that spot and make sure it's on for at least an hour. Then, when they insert the needle, you will not feel any pain, I swear. Pressure, but no pain at all. Awesome.

3. It pays to make nice to the lab nurses. They know all the good tricks and are a wealth of knowledge. If you get the same one most times, you can establish a routine. She'll know all the subtleties of your situation and what works for you. It helps to make these personal connections.

4. Check your shirt before you walk out of the lab. I got so blasé about the whole thing that I started to walk out into the waiting room with my shirt open

half the time. Seriously, I mean, after six months of unbuttoning my shirt for anyone who asked, who cares? Nothing to see here. Literally.

5. If you're squeamish about needles and things? Number one, I feel bad for you because the world you've now entered is filled with them. Number two, bring sunglasses and put them on when the needles come out. It's easier than trying not to look.

6. Okay, I know this is a "Top 6." It's truly odd, but you can sometimes taste the saline solution they use to flush the port. And, even odder, it doesn't taste like salt water, it tastes metallic. It's incomprehensible to me because the saline is going directly into the port, nowhere near my mouth. Bring a mint or a Tic Tac, and pop it in at the right time if it bothers you.

There are all sorts of things that people can be sensitive to, from the adhesives used to secure the tubing to the cleansing and sterilizing products. I found out that I was sensitive to predrawn saline solution from one distributor, so for a while they had to draw mine individually. I experienced a little stinging from it and mentioned to the nurse that I could feel it, and she switched and it made a huge difference. Not every nurse will mention your options, but some will. The trick is to mention everything you're feeling. Don't assume that things are supposed to sting or hurt or itch just because you're in a hospital getting treatment. Often the nurses know of something that will make things a little easier. Let's be clear: The whole thing sucks, and there will be lots of pain and discomfort along the way, but that's why little things can make such a big difference. Especially when it comes down to the nurses and your level of comfort with them. Everybody's different, so ask for the people you trust, and refuse the ones you don't. Nobody should ever make you feel guilty about it. You won't be the only one who has done this. I did.

The thing about lab work is that as unpleasant as it is, it's important. They're checking your blood levels to make sure you're okay to have treatment, so you have to go through it a lot. Each time is stressful because you're back in the oncology department, and anytime you're anywhere near that place, you're going to feel some anxiety. Add needles and flushes and treatments to that, and it's quite a package. Can't be helped. Remember that "new normal" everyone kept talking about? This is part of it.

5

Chemotherapy

DAY ONE

There are many different protocols and variations of treatment, but they all begin with the same question: What to wear? On the one hand—who cares? What a lousy day. You get up in the morning and you think, Oh my God, I'm actually going to have chemotherapy today. I'm all for cheerleading, and I'm a "Let's go fight!" kind of person, but every time I woke up from a fitful sleep on a chemo morning, my first thought was, I can't believe I have to do this. There was often an expletive to go with that. *Mostly* in my head. And the truth is, it's not that bad. Really. The actual experience of sitting in the chair is pretty much a nonevent most of the time. It's the idea of it and the side effects you know are coming, or that you worry are coming, that make it difficult on day one.

You do have to get dressed, though. You actually have to put on clothes and go to the clinic and have it all done to you. There's no way around it. It's the best treatment we have, and so we do it. We hate it, but we do it, and you will be able to handle it. The best thing to wear? Shirts that button or zip so there's easy access to your port, if you have one. If you don't, then anything that allows you comfortably to roll up the sleeve.

Make sure you start off right. Before you leave home, eat a real breakfast; you may not want to eat for the rest of the day. Even though you're already feeling sick to your stomach from nerves and anticipation, try to eat and drink something. You'll be given fluid through your IV, but you still don't want to be dehydrated, because that can make it difficult to access your port or start an IV. Being well hydrated helps the blood flow easier and more quickly.

Okay, so this is what really happens:

First you need to complete lab work. Have your blood drawn to check your red and white blood cell counts as well as your platelets. Your doctor needs to be sure you're well enough to get chemo. Then you review what's going to happen with your oncologist. Make sure you tell your doctor everything that's been going on since you saw her last. *Everything.* Make a list before you get to the hospital so that you don't forget anything (my husband and I used to put together my list on the drive over). Some of your issues may turn out to be side effects of sleeping pills, steroids, antianxiety meds, or something else. Don't be embarrassed, think it's insignificant, or assume it's not related. Sometimes you may just get a sympathetic nod, but you still need to mention all changes, whether physical or behavioral. Drugs of all kinds have side effects. Believe me, they can do strange things to you.

So now you're ready. Well, that's an exaggeration; you're never going to be ready for chemo. But let's assume your blood counts are fine, and now you go into that next waiting area. With your heart pounding, wearing your comfortable clothing, and tubing sticking out of you, they call your name and you go back to "the area." Chemo floors look about the same all over. In large hospitals there may be a few private rooms. In small clinics there may be rooms with two treatment chairs. There are often televisions, so you can catch up on the latest daytime drama, or reruns of *The Golden Girls*. In lots of settings there are reclining chairs lined up facing windows or one another, IV machines next to each one, and chairs for visitors. I always asked for a private room. If the wait was going to be too long, I took whatever I could get, but I liked the privacy because I always brought someone with me.

You sit down, and the nurse checks your name and birth date and sometimes asks for your weight, my least favorite part. You'd be surprised how many times you are weighed during this whole experience. *Every* time you see a doctor—which is a lot. (I may have only one boob, but I'm still a woman and I hate being weighed!)

If you've already been accessed for the lab work, you've got clear tubing sticking out of you. If not, then you have to be accessed again. When you sit down, the nurse will ask if you'd like a blanket or anything. I'm a big fan of blankets. Especially when they come preheated. Kind of like the hot towel in some restaurants—*sooo* nice.

Then you're done with prelims. All the nurses do is hang the see-through plastic sacks on the IV machine, plug the machine into your tubing, open the flow, and, voilà, it has begun! You may feel a little something in the catheter, but you can't feel the actual medicines. The first drugs they hook up are the premeds—antinausea drugs, steroids, and usually an antianxiety med like Ativan, which makes the antinausea drugs more effective. And they add a bag of saline solution as well. When the sacks of medicine are depleted, the machine beeps, and a nurse shows up to switch bags. When they start the actual chemo drugs, a second nurse comes in and checks that you are getting the correct meds. Sometimes the treatment is administered via a drip, sometimes as a "push," when the nurse uses a syringe to push the chemo into the catheter.

At this point you may feel sleepy from the pre-meds, or not. I never did.

You can unplug the machine and drag it to the bathroom so you're not confined for the whole time. The IV machines have battery backup so they still work.

If you feel anything peculiar at any time, tell someone! The way my port's catheter was positioned meant that I could feel the infusion starting through my veins. I'm just really sensitive, and the first time it freaked me out.

Oh boy did it *ever* freak me out! If you start out, as I did, on Adriamycin and Cytoxan (unfondly known as A/C), the first thing you learn about Adriamycin is how toxic it is. It's basically a type of poison designed to kill cancer, but it can kill lots of other things, too. And just to make sure you can't miss it, it's a vivid orange-red. There's a whole pamphlet about it, telling you how the nurse will administer this one by hand, and if you feel anything unusual, to let her know because it's really toxic to tissue. So I'm sitting there with my husband and mother, who are, of course, desperately trying to remain calm and cheerful while I start this grueling process, and I'm being hypervigilant. I thought that's what I was supposed to be. The nurse is pushing in this bright red fluid, and I'm thinking about it, and I feel something really weird. I tell the nurse, and she asks me what "weird" means. Can I describe it? Does it sting or burn, etc.? I start getting really anxious because I can't describe it. I mean, I never had anything like this before, and the sensation is in my neck, right where the catheter from my port is, and I'm just about hyperventilating, thinking that this toxic solution is leaking into my neck.

Of course I was totally fine, but my catheter turned out to be angled in such a way that I could actually feel things sliding through it. And that first time I was already anxious from having to start chemo and then trying to be my own advocate to the point of near hysteria. (My husband may suggest leaving out the "near.") Oh who cares? Starting chemo, you have the *right* to freak out. Although it really doesn't help matters much, and I'm here to tell you that it's really not that bad. Really. Have I said "really" enough to make you believe me yet?

Seriously, though, don't forget that you are already

doing about a million things that are awful. You don't need to put up with any more than you have to. And you don't need to be afraid to speak up. Be nice, but always speak up.

They tell you to meditate on the medicine that's going into your body and attacking the cancer cells. All I could think of was Pac-Man. So I pictured this bright orange–red stuff like a flaming Pac-Man, burning and eating the cancer cells. There's nothing to feel; it's just ugly to look at and very, very real.

After the poison they give you a little more saline, and maybe then a shot of Neulasta or Neupogen to boost your blood marrow production. This is another lovely treat—a shot right in the belly. Trick of the trade: The slower they push the plunger on the injection, the less it hurts. I learned this the hard way. The first nurse did it quick and dirty, and it hurt like hell. The second nurse took forever, and she even rubbed the skin with another finger while doing it, and it didn't hurt at all. I got her name and asked for her every week. Sometimes you might have to come back for the Neulasta shot on another day, or even give yourself one of these at home—I had the pleasure of experiencing all the options at one time or another. Apparently you may also be given this shot in the arm, but I got all mine in the belly.

WHAT TO BRING

Friends and/or family. Well, that's assuming you have friends or family who can be comforting and distracting (in a good way). You don't need anyone in the room adding to your stress. They can't put that on a prescription pad, but they should. You need people who are capable of being supportive and protective. I give bonus points for funny. Also, these rooms are small and not always private, so keep that in mind, too. My husband always came with me for the lab work and the meeting with the oncologist. He'd stay until I was hooked up, and then my mom or one of my friends would take over and keep me entertained during treatments. I was lucky to have people willing to come with me every week, and it made the time pass. Even with TVs in the room and an iPad, I always found that time moved faster when I had company. It's really not scary for someone to watch, so if you have friends who are willing to accompany you, take them up on their offers. If you can, have people come more than once. The second time is more familiar, more comfortable for them. Also, once they've learned the routine, they might notice if something seems unusual.

Do not let anyone come who might be overly emotional or a burden. This is not the place for that. Your chemo buddy's job is to make you feel better and pass the time. It's not your job to reassure anyone that you're okay.

I always brought a cozy blanket with me. All hospitals have warm blankets, but I also liked having my own. Some hospitals have a room with snacks and drinks, and I suggest you check it out during your first visit. If you don't like what they offer, bring your own because the hospital's selection will never change. I couldn't eat during chemo, but some people can, so it pays to have things you like around in case you're hungry.

You will quickly learn which nurses are the most competent and which are the least. Ask for the nurses who are best for you and make you feel the most comfortable. A day in chemo is stressful enough, and a less than excellent nurse can make it worse. Make a note of the names of the nurses you like and those you don't, and when you check in, ask for the ones you like and never take one you don't. Just quietly mention that you'd be more comfortable with someone else. You don't have to explain yourself, although you may have to wait another minute or two if your favorite nurse is busy. It's worth the wait. You will not be the only one doing this, I promise. You're going through hell; take comfort where you can!

TOP 5 TIPS DURING CHEMO

1. Drink ice water and suck on ice chips or Popsicles (you can bring them in a cooler) during chemo. It helps prevent mouth sores.

2. If you have to go back in for a Neulasta shot, or give one to yourself (like I did), take a Claritin or Zyrtec starting twenty-four hours before the shot. Somehow it helps counteract bone pain, which can follow. Not every doctor will mention this, so be sure to ask if yours doesn't talk about it.

3. Bring only the people with whom you feel totally comfortable. This is one of the most vulnerable periods of your life, and you need to feel supported. You should feel free to be pathetic and whiny, strong and funny, sleepy, famished, frightened—any or all of them. This is not the time to put on a show. Or a wig, or a boob, for that matter, if you don't feel like it. Be as comfortable as you can. It is also okay if you want to go it alone (although I do not recommend this for the first chemo appointment). If you are not up for sharing the experience with anyone, that's fine. The mantra here is do whatever you makes you the most comfortable.

4. Plan for extra time. Remember, this is health care; things often take longer than you think—especially the first time. Ask your doctor how long it should take, and then add an hour just to be certain. You don't want the person who's supposed to be driving you home looking at her watch and asking you how much longer it will be. Yes, this very thing actually happened to someone I know. As if the patient should keep a tighter schedule!

5. Use the EMLA cream at least an hour before your port is accessed to numb the site.

THE CHEMO ROOM

What does it feel like to be sitting in that chair? In the beginning it's dreadful. Not that you're being tortured, because you're not—you're being saved, actually—but the whole thing and the idea of what's happening to you is just plain awful. It's stressful to worry about all the medications and side effects, and if you've recently had a mastectomy, you're still dealing with a lot of pain.

Believe it or not, it does become more or less routine. After a while, you know the staff, they know your needs, and it's not quite as bad. But I did find that every Tuesday morning I had trouble getting dressed. I just hated getting dressed for chemo. Somehow I felt as if I shouldn't have to be dressed at all. I wished I could just go in my pajamas, but it wasn't my style. Getting up and ready on those days was really hard. Go in your pj's if it makes you feel better. I didn't actually see anyone in giant footy pajamas, but it would have made me smile if I had.

You've heard the stories of the women who go to chemo in their Prada and Chanel. I saw *Sex and the City*. I have to tell you, don't feel pressured by those women. Again, do what you feel most comfortable doing. Chemo isn't a time to feel social pressure to be fabulous and fun. Be fair to yourself instead. If you're a Samantha, embrace it. But if you're an Andrea (that's me), then couture and chemo don't mix.

Finally it's over—after hours and hours—and they pull the tubing out of your arm or port and send you home with a Band-Aid covering the spot. I always found it somewhat ironic that the whole thing ends with a Band-Aid. I think they should at least have superhero or Dora the Explorer ones. Kind of reminds me of when my kids were little, and they wanted a Band-Aid on everything. Like they were magic. Here's hoping.

It doesn't hurt when they take the needle out, just a click and a tug. You will be exhausted mentally and physically; it's draining. But on the day of chemo, you will probably just feel tired from the stress and from some of the antinausea and antianxiety drugs. The side effects don't kick in for a day or two or three. Everyone's different, and you'll learn your own pattern, but for most people it's around the third day after chemo. So if you're working, try to schedule your infusions for a Tuesday or Wednesday so you can be home on the weekend. Make a note the first week when your worst symptoms kick in, so you can organize your schedule.

After chemo you always go home to your giant collection of pill bottles. There are antianxiety, antinausea, antibiotics, antacids, stool softeners, pain medications, sleep aids—just about everything you could possibly think of, and then some. It's amazing how much a little nightstand can hold.

I really can't go any further without talking about the ticking time bomb that has just started. The bald bomb. Some of the new targeting therapies do not make your hair fall out, but many chemo agents either make the hair thin or fall out completely. I know this is not news to you, and it's one of the biggest concerns women have when learning they have breast cancer. Some of most common chemotherapy drugs and their effect on your hair are:

- Cytoxan (cyclophosphamide) causes hair thinning but not complete hair loss.
- Adrucil (fluorouracil) does not cause hair loss.
- Adriamycin (doxorubicin) causes hair to thin during the first three weeks of treatment; then all the hair falls out.
- Taxol (paclitaxel) causes very sudden hair loss.

All you've ever wanted to know about going and being bald is in the next chapter, so feel free to skip ahead.

In the beginning I decided the one place I really didn't want to wear a wig was during chemo. I later changed my mind, but in the beginning it just felt like one thing too many to deal with so I mostly wore scarves to treatment. Each one made me feel like a different version of myself. My mom gave me a really beautiful red-and-black one I wore one day, and it made me feel like I was going to a poetry reading at a coffeehouse instead of being Chemo Girl. Neat trick.

The first chemo treatment is emotionally draining because you don't know what to expect. The second is still exhausting. I came home and crashed for at least an hour right after my second treatment. Didn't hear anyone come to the door, didn't hear the phone ring. Nothing. Woke up feeling . . . wonky. A little headachy, a little bit nauseous, but no big deal. Just like the first time. I sat around writing in a Snuggie. Just like the TV commercials. You can write, work, watch TV. Mom gave it to me. So, all in all, the first couple of treatments can be just that simple.

TOP 5 TIPS AFTER CHEMO

∽

1. Have a little notebook or datebook that's for listing medications and their doses, along with when you're supposed to take them. They seem to change almost weekly, and sometimes it's hard to keep track. You might also want to use the notebook to keep notes on all your doctor and treatment appointments.

2. Take a permanent marker and write the name and dose of the medicine right on the top of the bottle cap in big letters. It's really hard to read the label on each bottle, especially when there are generic

---

names on them. On some I even drew pictures to remind me which was which—that is, a smiley face for antianxiety, and so on. This is one time in your life when you want easy access to drugs!

3. Drink lots of water. You can become dehydrated before you know it, and everything is worse if you're dehydrated. Drink before, during, and after chemo. Then drink some more.

4. Take a walk afterward. Yes, drag your sorry self around the block for at least ten or fifteen minutes after your treatment. This tip should really have a big star next to it. My physical therapist would be so proud. This is one of the harder things to do, but it makes a huge difference in how you will feel later. Walking every day, but especially on treatment day, gets the poison moving through your body and out again. It reminds your healthy cells what they're supposed to be doing, and oxygenating your body is extremely important during chemotherapy. I enlisted whoever drove me home from chemo to walk with me, too. Coming to chemo with me meant bringing your walking shoes.

5. Take the drugs! Take the drugs! Did I mention you should take the drugs?! Almost every single person

I spoke to who had a hard time with nausea started out by saying, "Well, I didn't take everything they gave me right away." Hello, anybody home? I'm sorry, but take the freaking medicine! You just had a course of chemotherapy, some of the strongest drugs you'll ever take, so let's not quibble about the ones that are actually supposed to help you feel better. If you stay ahead of it, you'll do fine. If you wait until you feel sick, you'll spend the next half day trying to catch up. It's *so* not worth it. I don't know if this is when people decide they need to take control of what happens to them, and so they hold back, or whether it's some sort of martyr thing, but *take the drugs*! Of course, I didn't have natural childbirth either, so feel free to dismiss my opinion.

THE SIDE EFFECTS

They don't kick in right away, and they change all the time. I had most of them.

Nausea is the one everyone wants to know about. Are you hanging on to the toilet, vomiting? Not usually. The antinausea drugs they give you as premeds during the infusion and the oral ones you take when you get home *do* work. But you have to take them as prescribed. Don't wait until you feel sick; it's too late by then. If yours don't work, tell your doctor immediately so you can try something else. You really don't need to feel horribly nauseated on chemo. It's manageable. That's not to say that you will feel entirely well, either. It's something in between. Are you picturing being on the bathroom floor every day? It doesn't work like that. The antinausea drugs make it more like waves of wooziness that come and go. You have a few hours of energy, then feel the need to lie down. Then you get up and do it all over again. The physical sensation I got wasn't exactly nausea. I called it "feeling wonky." It wasn't that I thought I was going to throw up all the time (although I did occasionally do that as well); it was just that I didn't feel at all right when it came to thinking about, looking at, or smelling food.

After the first couple of treatments you will begin to understand what "cumulative" means as far as side effects. The fatigue seems a little deeper each week, and it seems like almost every day there's a new and exciting physical experience. Toward the end of chemo treatments that cumulative thing really starts to kick in. Remember, everyone has slightly different reactions to the drugs, and having some complications is completely normal and expected. I had my complications a month after I started treatments, and I woke up with every muscle in my body aching— get this—including my eyes! Seriously, my eyes hurt. How weird is that? And some other side effects you need not know about. I took Ambien and got a few hours' sleep and woke up still with the eye pain. Called the doctor in the morning, and the nurse said, "Wow, that's a weird one, but don't worry." Just what you want to hear, right?

She did say it was nothing to worry about, just unfortunate. Your body just has strange reactions to the drugs, and you just never know. It's probably muscle pain, a common side effect, but for some reason it had affected my eye muscles (I'm so special).

If you are really ill after chemo, tell your doctor and keep at him until he finds a combination of drugs that works for you. You may need a slightly different cocktail, and there are many to try. This will not be as much fun as sampling cocktails at the local bar, but it may be necessary. Some of the best ones are also the most expensive, so he'll often try the cheapest first to see if they work for you. This is all I will say about the insurance portion of my experience. I could write a whole book on billing and medical coverage. Actually, I couldn't because I don't understand it.

Back to our regularly scheduled programming.

For the first eight weeks on chemo, I pretty much lost my appetite. This was a bizarre thing for me because I am a foodie. I *love* food, *live* for chocolate, and normally spend all day thinking about where my next meal is coming from. To all of a sudden forget to eat, have no desire for chocolate, and be completely turned off by food was a truly unique experience.

I did have some real aversions. Seafood in particular. This is a common one. And anything spicy. All I wanted was comfort food. Mashed potatoes, ice cream, etc. I never even liked mashed potatoes before, but when your taste buds go completely bonkers, it's easier to eat something that you know doesn't taste like much, rather than something you expect to taste a certain way; then, when you put it in your mouth, it's all wrong. I couldn't even talk about food for those eight weeks. Literally. My friends would sign up to bring dinner for my family and call to ask what I wanted, and if they started to describe the food, I'd have to hand the phone to my wonderful mother, who would say something kind like, "Andrea's just going to go lie down now. Can I help?" She was awesome.

I know that some people gain weight on chemo, especially if they're on steroids, but I lost about fifteen pounds. That was the best part of the whole experience! And if it happens, you'll know it, because they weigh you every week. My entire married life (eighteen years) I had never told my husband how much I weighed. Now every week he knew. Ah, the indignities! As if the scars and treatment weren't enough—now he has to know what I weigh! I won't even get started on all the advice I received about what I should and shouldn't eat. Remember: Ignore any advice that doesn't come from your doctor or another established source. Just smile and say thank you. Note that there's some recent information about too many antioxidants interfering with chemo, so beware the berry pushers.

I started chemo with eight weeks of A/C. Then, after a three-week break, I began a different chemo regimen.

More Top 5s—you need a few extra Top 5s for chemo:

TOP 5 TIPS FOR HANDLING CHEMO

∞

1. Did I say take the meds? Your oncologist will probably offer you a buffet of antinausea medication.

Read all the labels and call the office if you need to add on. I had a Chinese menu of drugs some days. One from column A, one from column B: Compazine, Kytril, EMEND—the list goes on. Put food in your stomach every few hours, even if you have to set an alarm to make yourself do it. Saltines, organic apples, anything you can tolerate. The less acid buildup in your stomach, the better. Beware of tomatoes and anything with a high acidic content. They may cause mouth sores. If you have a craving, try rinsing your mouth out immediately after eating. Some say it helps.

2. Mouth sores. Nearly everybody gets them. Two types of prescription medicines may help. The first is a cream you put directly on the sores (triamcinolone acetonide dental paste). The second is a mouthwash with lidocaine in it, a BMX cocktail (Benadryl, lidocaine viscous, and Maalox). The mouthwash completely numbs your mouth, so it helps with the pain, but it really does numb your whole mouth. Try using a Q-tip to dab it only on the spots that hurt, so you don't act like you've just come from a major root canal. The first time I used it, I just followed the directions and dribbled all over

myself when I tried to drink. It was hilarious. You can also ask your doctor about lysine. It is an amino acid and is available in several different forms, and it has been shown to be effective in reducing the frequency of mouth sores.

3. Keep exercising all the way through chemo. Even if it's just a walk around the block some days. I went to physical therapy during chemo as part of the wellness program for cancer patients at my hospital (check your options at your medical facility). I didn't realize how important physical therapy can be in helping patients deal with the side effects of chemo. I thought it was just about healing from surgery. They may teach you how to exercise, when, how much, which days, and so on. All having to do with one's own body's responses to treatment. It's not about being fit or getting stronger, it's about minimizing the effects of chemotherapy and cancer on your body.

Of course they all told me I was just the perfect patient. The poster child for wellness. They all acted surprised when I could do all the range of motion exercises and that I was walking twenty to forty minutes a day. I told them I read the pamphlet. It's not rocket science. Even the poster child for wellness had to cancel all afternoon plans occasionally and take a nap, though, so don't push yourself too hard.

4. Be kind to yourself. What you're going through is really tough. Stick with it. There is an end in sight. Forgive yourself if you can't walk one day or do all the exercises. Just be sure to try the next day.

5. Drink plenty of water. Filtered or bottled, of course. You're immune system is challenged enough right now.

COMPLICATIONS— AND MORE SIDE EFFECTS

There are *always* complications. Maybe the drain from the mastectomy gets infected. Maybe your port doesn't work one day. Maybe you're allergic to one of the drugs. Maybe your blood counts get too low. The truth is that nobody goes through the whole process smoothly. People have all sorts of complications. Most are expected, but even the unexpected can be dealt with.

One day in December I woke up completely drained and looking gray. After my slight meltdown, which included tears when I couldn't locate the shirt I was planning to wear, with the buttons that make it easy to access my port, Richard and I finally made our way to the hospital—where they couldn't access my port. They tried everything and then had to give me the enzyme again, and this time said I had to wait two hours. In the meantime I told them just to take it out of my left arm so they could run the blood work.

We went to see my oncologist, who, along with the nurse, was quite taken aback at how I looked. They did a thorough exam, listened to my lungs, went over all the side effects, and decided that I was allergic to Taxol and needed to be on Abraxane for the rest of my treatment. It's a related but different formulation, with none of the allergic issues. It's also the one used for metastatic breast cancer. I asked if it's so much easier to tolerate, why doesn't everyone get it? Turns out most people do tolerate Taxol very well, and of those who don't, almost all have a reaction during the first infusion. My prolonged reactions were very rare. See, I told you I'm special. It's also thirty—yes, thirty—times more expensive than Taxol, and there's no generic. See, I'm even more special—I'm *platinum* special!

Then the nurse walked in with my blood count results, and everyone's mood changed. Very, very,

very low. They sent me for a chest X-ray and decided I would get IV antibiotics and fluids, and then just Herceptin, because my counts were too low for any other chemotherapy. As I walked out to get the chest X-ray, the office staff asked whether Andrea needed a wheelchair. Yes, that's how bad I looked. I got upstairs for the X-ray, which turned out to be fine. Nothing to find, which meant I had an irritation of the lungs caused by Taxol.

We made it into the chemo area, and they accessed my port. No problem, whoopee! I figured things were turning around. They started me on saline solution and then the IV antibiotic. After twenty minutes, the second nurse came in and discovered that the first had not actually turned on the antibiotic flow, so we were now thirty minutes behind. Okay, no worries, we had nowhere to be.

Then we were cooking along for a while, so I decided to take a potty break. I noticed that the skin around my nose and mouth was starting to get very red. Okay . . . My friend who was with me said she just noticed this as well. We called in the nurse (the second one, as the first one had not noticed). She said she didn't like that at all and called my oncologist, who came down to look. They decided I was having another reaction, and they added an IV steroid to the list of meds I was going to get. That would take another thirty minutes. Okay, still no place to go. Then my tongue started to feel funny. Are you getting the pattern? Then my cheeks started to turn red. My oncologist continued to visit periodically. They added Benadryl and a codeine cough syrup for my cough. Tick-tock. It was decided that unless these reactions calmed down, there would be no Herceptin that day. My body wouldn't be able to take it.

Long story short. The long story is: Eight hours later my friend Bobbie was finally able to go home! What a trouper. She had made me laugh, and we talked all day. We did watch one video: *How to Give Yourself a Subcutaneous Injection*. I had to give myself injections three times a week to pump up my blood counts. I managed. It's that first jab that's tough.

I'm one of the three percent of people who had a severe reaction to all forms of Taxol. And not the kind of reaction that they warn you about where the symptoms appear in the office. Mine evolved over a ten-day period; every day a new and strange symptom popped up.

My eyes hurt, like when you have a fever, only way worse, and they turned red. The tops of my fingers (from the last knuckle up) turned red and swelled and hurt, then later blistered. I had to soak them in ice water in the middle of the night. Cracking, red, and peeling fingers and fingernails are actually a relatively common side effect of chemo, but mine included bright redness and pain. On top of it I had a severe reaction to the second chemo drug, Herceptin, which put me in the hospital for two weeks. These things are rare, but they happen. And yet I'm still here, writing this book. My point is that you are going to go through some pretty complex experiences with this complex disease. Everybody responds differently. Often your doctor or nurse may seem surprised, or mention that a certain reaction is unusual. Don't worry when they say that. It is all about managing expectations. Your doctors will paint as positive a picture as they can for you and hope that it all goes like clockwork. It rarely does. That clock has a way of stopping and starting and skipping ahead. It's part of medicine. There are always unforeseen events, and you have to go through the process of figuring it all out. As the bumper sticker says, "Stuff happens." Well, you know what the bumper sticker actually says.

My body felt like it had been abducted by aliens. Not the cute E.T. ones, either—the ones who perform experiments on you to learn about humans. This feeling passes, eventually. My husband just kept reminding me that it was all due to the drugs. And when chemo was over, this stuff would be gone. Of course, we didn't say "stuff."

HOT FLASHES

First of all, hot flashes are not just hot flashes, they are prickles and tingles followed by flop sweat followed by cold flashes. One time I sweated so much my wig nearly slipped off my head. I ran to powder rooms all over Seattle to rip off my wig and let my scalp air-dry for a minute. Although these hot flashes are technically the same as those that women get with menopause, I've been told they're more intense and occur more often with chemo.

I had to take my wig in to replace the wig tape with elastic because I was sweating so much during my hot flashes that the wig tape wouldn't stick. Besides, I really needed to be able to whip my wig on and off at a moment's notice to regulate my body temperature. Of course I only performed this act in the privacy of my bedroom or a locked bathroom stall, but it was necessary. I'm not sure why they're called hot flashes. You're only hot for a few minutes, then freezing cold. It's really just a constant tipping of the scale twenty-four hours a day. Layers on—layers off.

Here's my own personal list of weird side effects,
from the uncomfortable to the downright painful:

1. Fingers blistering and peeling from Taxol. The skin at
   the tips of my fingers turned red, then blistered, then
   peeled. Remember, though, this is a common side
   effect and not an indication of an allergic reaction.

2. Nail changes. *Nail changes?!* That's what they were
   called in the guide to chemotherapy that the hospital gave me. What this means is that your nails may
   stop growing, like your hair, then separate from the
   skin. Yes, separate. This is not fun. First, your fingers get really sensitive because of the separation.
   And then, as the nail starts to grow again, eventually they get to a certain point where the old nails
   fall off, and you're left with a teeny spot of nail and
   a very sensitive exposed fingertip. I have no advice
   for this. I tried Krazy Glue, like you do when you
   break a nail, but it didn't really help. When the nails
   are growing and start to look normal on the top,
   sometimes a layer of dead or damaged nail is still
   underneath the new, healthy nail. I kept trying to
   clean it out. Eventually they grow in normally, and
   you can just trim that part off.

3. Numbness, pains, and itching. The surgical site is numb to the touch, but there are still big pains and little pains and itches that occur, and you just can't get to them. You know what it feels like to deal with numbness from trips to the dentist and when your leg falls asleep? It's kind of like that—with the lovely advantage of never going away permanently. They come and go. You get used to it.

4. Painful eyes. My eyeballs got painful, but that was a bizarre allergic reaction, so I hope nobody else gets that. In case you do—you're not alone!

5. I broke out in an itchy rash on my hands. It was bad, and nothing they told me to try worked, so I ended up using the magic mouth-sore mouthwash (the Benadryl/Lidocaine/Maalox cocktail) on my hands. Guess what? It worked! I smelled like Maalox, but who cares!

6. Neuropathy. Okay, this is actually sharp, intense pain. I am sorry, but nobody explained this to me, so I'm telling you right now. Chemo neuropathy basically means that the nerves, usually to your hands and feet, have been damaged by the drugs. It feels like shooting or searing or pricking pains in your hands and/or feet. This *is* temporary, but it

really sucks! The treatment options for neuropathy are vitamins, especially B vitamins (B_1, B_6, and B_{12}). The treatments for other side effects are gentle laxatives for constipation, prescribed medication such as steroids, lidocaine patches, capsaicin creams, antidepressants, antiseizure medications, and pain medications.

7. Fatigue. This is real. It's draining. It's cumulative. It feels like you're wearing a lead suit some days. It comes on after a few treatments. At some point in almost every day I felt as if the plug had been pulled out of the bathtub, and all the energy just drained out. I would have to lie down and nap, but I'd wake up feeling not much better.

I went a few times to a therapist who specializes in cancer patients (more on that later), and the first time I went I was in the waiting room wearing my white cotton gloves to protect and heal the still-cracked and healing fingers. So of course everyone who walked in stared at my hands, thinking I must be some sort of germophobe or Michael Jackson fanatic. The psychiatrist also took a quick peek as she ushered me in. I debated whether to say anything, because I was going to see how long it took her to ask, but I figured I didn't want to waste my time, so I explained right away. She said, "I did notice. I'm glad we don't have to spend time on that. Actually that tells me that you're willing to do whatever it takes to beat this disease, and that's that." She got me.

Just like in your pre-cancer life (if you can re-member it), you're going to have good days and bad. During my treatment I wrote a blog on www.caring bridge.org to keep all my friends and family abreast (sorry) of my situation, and here are two entries that show just how far you can sway in a few weeks:

End of December

Went to the hospital today and saw the doctor
in charge of my physical therapy program.
We discussed the pain in my arm and fatigue
management. I declined medication for my arm
pain. It's bearable, and I'm trying to limit the
number of pills I'm taking to about 100/day.
He says I'm a "wonder." I say he says that to
all the girls. He says that because I can stand up
and smile this week that qualifies me for being a
wonder. I say he should have higher standards.
Seriously, though, many people at this point in

their treatment, after the last A/C, are completely worn out. I'm doing ok. I'm tired for sure, but I can still function. Most of the time.

Actually I think it's a combination of doing what I'm told by the doctors as far as eating and exercising (even on days when I just want to stay in bed), lucky reaction to the drugs, and my great network of support.

January 24

I am a slug. I am not embarrassed to say that I put my pajamas on at 5 p.m.

Today's boo-boo (you thought I was going to say "boob," didn't you?) report:

1. *chemo nose*

2. *mouth sores*

3. *scary article about breast cancer in the* New York Times

4. *ticklish throat*

5. *completely exhausted from having about an hour (total) of sleep last night*

6. *hard to know if you're getting a cold when you have #1.*

TOP 5 TIPS FOR DEALING
WITH SIDE EFFECTS

1. Check the listed side effects for all the drugs you're taking—for anxiety, sleep, whatever—because some include things that you may think are normal, like hot flashes; but if your drug-caused hot flashes really are interfering in your life, you might want to change drugs. When I say check the list of side effects, I mean check the whole list. Read all the way to the bottom. I turned out to be a bottom-dweller; you just never know.

2. This tip came from my wonderful oncologist, Dr. Erin Ellis: Get some Bag Balm, the stuff in the green tin, and cosmetic gloves. They don't have to be the high-end kind; lots of drugstores sell cheaper ones. Slather the balm on your hands, and keep the gloves on. It made a *huge* difference. Same goes for your feet, but for them you can just use cotton socks.

3. When your numb spots itch, around the mastectomy scar, for instance, scratch anyway. I have no scientific proof for this, but I think your brain knows

you're scratching the area, and so sometimes it
helps. So does distraction. Do something physical
to distract yourself from the sensation.

4. Be on the alert, but try not to be obsessed by every
ache and pain and odd sensation. This is a balanc-
ing act, and it's really hard. How can you not be
paranoid? But don't be paranoid.

5. My doctor told me to take vitamin B_6 for my neuropathy. It seemed to help me. You should check
with your doctor to see if it might help you.

STEROIDS

Chances are if you are having chemo, you will be on
steroids for at least part of your treatment. They prevent inflammatory reactions to the drugs you're taking. And they are necessary and amazing. And you and
your family will *hate* them. There is a term in chemo-
land called "steroid rage." This is the uncontrollable,
head-spinning, earsplitting, tear-inducing, screaming
fit of anger you may perhaps experience every three to
five days. And there is nothing you or anyone else can
do about it. My daughter called me "Steroid Mommy"

and would look to her father for confirmation that I had gone crazy when I would lose it at the dinner table because of some imagined insult and ground her for the rest of her life. My husband would stare like a deer in the headlights, not knowing which way to turn. On the one hand he had an obviously jacked-up and overreacting wife who would tear him limb from limb should he side with his clearly wronged daughter. On the other he faced the wrath of a very right teenage daughter. Run, run for the hills!

I, of course, had no idea what the big deal was. I mean, maybe I was just a tad sensitive on Fridays, but certainly not nickname-worthy, right? *Wrong.* As the weeks wore on I would occasionally become aware of a banshee screaming in my ear. I would turn to see who could be speaking in such a caustic tone, and I would find myself face to face with *me.* Once I said to my husband, "Sometimes I plan what I'm going to say, and how I'm going to say it. And then I listen to what comes out of my mouth, and it bears no relation at all to what I'd planned." You just have to keep reminding your family about the steroids and beg forgiveness. And maybe find a soundproof room to lock yourself in every once in a while. Try to note which day this starts to happen, so you (and they) can be prepared with headphones, a rope to tie you down, and a hotel room to run to. This, too, shall pass.

This slightly-out-of-control feeling went on for a while. Then, when I had my very rare reaction to Herceptin, they had to put me on a whopping dose of steroids. Good news—in two hours I felt better. Bad news—even bigger mood swings and steroid withdrawal from an even higher dose. Stepping down from this was more like falling off a cliff. My back hurt as if I'd been hit by a truck. I got the shakes and chills and was a complete wreck. The bigger the dose, the bigger the fall. I fell off that cliff for thirty hours.

TOP TIP FOR STEROID SIDE EFFECTS—YUP, ONLY ONE PIECE OF ADVICE FOR STEROID POPPERS

1. Understand that you are not in control of yourself at some moments and forgive yourself; and remind your family and friends that it's the drugs doing the talking.

DRUG ALLERGIES AND ADVERSE REACTIONS—WHAT ABRAXANE DID FOR ME

The good news is that if you're allergic to Taxol, your doctor can put you on Abraxane. Abraxane has been known to have far fewer side effects. "Fewer" doesn't mean "none." I was so relieved that there was something else I could take that I didn't focus on what those fewer side effects might be. That is, until my fingernails started to bruise. I noticed my fingertips were extremely painful, and then I realized that my fingernails were breaking down almost to the cuticle. Some of them actually became black and blue, and the rest kind of red. The tops started to crack off. Seriously, as if losing my hair and eyelashes and most of my eyebrows wasn't bad enough, now I'm losing my fingernails, too? It happened on my big toes as well. Maybe the little toenails are too small to be affected, but *ouch*! I could barely text or type for weeks. Nobody, and I mean nobody, ever mentioned this lovely possibility to me. The good news—like my hair, my nails started to grow back. The bad news—short of wearing those white gloves all day, I couldn't hide it. They don't make wigs for your nails, and you can't put polish on them because supposedly it can weaken them even more. Lovely.

Chemotherapy in all its forms is, of course, the most dreaded treatment. Your oncologist is going to put you on the regimen she thinks is the best way to save your life, but that doesn't mean you shouldn't ask questions.

TOP 5 TIPS FOR UNDERSTANDING YOUR TREATMENTS

∞

1. Make sure you understand your particular course of treatment. What drugs you'll be on and for how long. Write it down. Bring someone to the appointments who can take notes and help you remember.

2. Make sure you understand why your doctor has chosen your particular sequence of chemo. There aren't unlimited options, but there are a few, and you should know how your doctor chose yours.

3. Don't be scared if things go awry. They often do. These are very powerful drugs, and they're not yet refined to the point that they target only cancer cells. That's why your hair falls out. Even if you have to postpone treatment for a little while to raise your white counts, or recover from a reaction, as long as

---

you come back to it you're still getting profound benefits from the drugs.

4. Give yourself a break. Chemo takes a lot out of you. When your white counts are down because your body is fighting the cancer and the effects of the chemo, you'll feel fatigued and sometimes tearful. It's all part of the side effects. You will rebound and not be a crying mess forever. I can't tell you how many women have come into our support group, every one of them in about the same phase of chemo (around cycle 4), crying and feeling like they'll never stop and be strong again. A few weeks later Wonder Woman returns, gold power bracelets flashing and ready to take on the world.

5. Don't worry if you are following a different protocol than other people you know. There are quite a few different treatment protocols, depending on your exact type of cancer, size of tumor, stage, oncotype, and even lifestyle. Once you understand why your doctor has chosen your protocol, feel free to get a second opinion if you have any lingering doubts about it.

6

Bald Is Better with Earrings

I'm wondering how many of you skipped right to this section.

How and when to shave your head—and then what?

First of all, I need to be honest. I never, ever got comfortable looking at myself bald. Many women I spoke to did, and many more did not. I dreaded losing my hair even more than losing a breast. Even though only one grows back. I had fabulous, long thick hair that people always remarked on. The kind of hair that the shampoo girls at the salon always said, "Wow. You have such great hair!" And I'd had it at least shoulder length since I was sixteen. I wasn't vain about it. I didn't spend hours curling or straightening or anything. But still, as for many women, my hair was a huge part of how I saw myself when I looked in the mirror.

So when I knew I was having chemo, and I knew I was going to lose my hair, I did a ton of research and read everything I could find. I talked to everyone about what they did and when and how, and how it felt. Even after all that there were things I still had to learn myself.

Everyone's entitled to a good cry now and then, and for many of us, after the shock of the diagnosis, the next cry is all about the hair. My mom says she takes full responsibility for the fact that I'm traumatized about shaving my head because when I was six years old, she had all my hair cut off and I looked like a boy. I never got over it, and that's why I've had long hair ever since! Of course, she still maintains that I looked adorable, but . . . My dad offered to shave his head in sympathy, but really, nobody wanted to see that, right? Nice, though. I walked around the night before they were going to shave my head with one of my oh-so-pretty headscarves purchased just for Chemo Girl and tried to get used to the view.

The number one thing to know: If you are on Adriamycin or Taxol in chemotherapy, your hair *will* fall out—100 percent of the time. It starts to happen just after the second week. Around day twelve. Like clockwork, so set your alarm. It's actually not really 100 percent of your hair, but it may as well be.

You will be essentially completely bald, even though some hairs stick around. Unfortunately those may be 1 percent or less of all the hair on your head. Even for a head of hair like mine, this is the equivalent of being bald, but in fact you don't go completely bald. It's more like a Dr. Seuss character. Bald head with ten hairs sticking straight up. So, you will have to decide . . .

TO SHAVE OR NOT TO SHAVE

Without exception, every single woman I talked to recommended that I shave my hair off *before* the chemo made it start falling out. Including many women who had waited until theirs did start falling out. Of those, almost all said they waited because they just couldn't bear the thought of shaving their heads, but then the actual experience of clumps of hair falling out unexpectedly was far more traumatic than shaving would have been.

I was fortunate to live in Bellevue, Washington, where one of the last great hair artists lives. Anton and his son, Kurt, make wigs out of your own hair. This is not cheap, but for me (and as a gift from my parents), it was a godsend. More on this in the wig section. So for me it was Kurt who shaved my head.

I brought my two best girlfriends, and they brought champagne (which we did not drink because I didn't exactly feel like celebrating, but I wish I had) and chocolate (which we ate, and I'm glad I did).

When Kurt shaved my head, he left about three-quarters of an inch all around, and one thing I did not expect was how gray I was! I'd been coloring my hair for years, and now the roots were exposed. I think this turned out for the best, because now I knew what to expect when it started to grow back, but it was shocking. If you've been coloring your hair for years, be warned: You will now see how gray you really are. Either now, or when it starts to grow back.

Another thing I was surprised about was how different my head felt. How much lighter (good) and also how much more sensitive (bad). When you're used to a protective coating of hair on your scalp, being newly shorn is *very* different. It does make for a good transition, though, to go from medium or long hair to short before heading straight to cue ball.

HAIR TODAY, GONE TOMORROW

Then the little bit that is left starts to fall out. It really does, and it's not fun. It doesn't fall out in one day, but it is pretty dramatic when it happens. Everyone I talked to felt the same need I did, to pull and rub and get them all out when it starts. It's cathartic somehow, like scratching an itch. I even took one of those lint catchers that's like a giant roll of masking tape and rolled that up and down my scalp. It takes a few days or a week. Even then there will be some stubborn hairs left. That's when I shaved with an electric razor, so I could be more comfortable. *Warning*: If you're Caucasian, your scalp will be *really white*. Especially if you have thick hair. It's very different from a man going bald over time. Your scalp has most likely not been exposed since you were an infant, so be prepared for the extreme whiteness: It's dramatic.

TOP 5 TIPS FOR WHEN YOU ARE GOING BALD

1. Start shaving from the back and move forward. It's far less traumatic that way. In the movies they always start at the front, and you've seen how that goes. Professionals start in the back.

2. Leave a little bit of a buzz cut that first time, because those hairs actually need to fall out to avoid leaving little bumps on your head. Leave about

three-quarters to one inch of a tag so they will fall out comfortably.

3. Have a wig ready and waiting. Even if you ultimately decide not to wear a wig, I recommend you have one on hand just in case. You may think you'll be fine without one and then change your mind when you first see yourself bald. On the other hand, you may think you'll never go without a wig, and decide you prefer yourself bald. I actually ended up with a few wigs, and I named them. The first was made of my own hair, so I called it Andrea. The second was a long redhead, and she was Fifi, of course, and the third was a cute short and sassy number I named Jackie. I wore them according to my mood and activity. For example, I never wore Fifi to chemo. It just didn't seem right to take her there.

4. Get a little cap to sleep in. It will make you feel more comfortable on the pillow and keep your head warm. And if you're really traumatized, you will avoid the shock of getting up in the middle of the night and seeing yourself bald.

5. Get some Aveda Men Pure-Formance exfoliating shampoo. Right, it's for men. This was a trick I learned from another survivor. One tube will last

you the whole experience, but it's the only shampoo I found that feels good on a bald head. It also
protects your scalp from those ingrown hairs, and
it smells good.

Yes, my eyelashes fell out, too, but not until the very end of all my chemo treatments. That really does make you look odd. It's amazing what that little line of lashes does to define your eye, even if they're really short. This was when people started asking me how I felt. It's about the same time that your skin gets that horrible chemo pallor, and then you have no eyelashes, and you just plain look like a cancer patient. Makeup helps, but I just couldn't be bothered most of the time, and when you don't have eyelashes, your eyes can really become irritated. After all, the lashes are there to keep dust and debris from entering the eye. I started to remember ninth-grade human biology around this time. My eyes got red and teary quite often. I was fortunate not to lose my eyebrows completely, but they did thin. If this really bothers you, of course you can draw them in. If you lose them completely, there are fake eyebrows you can glue on, just like fake eyelashes. They're pretty good, too; just search online.

Same goes for pubic hair. Not that there's glue-on for that. Well, maybe there is, but I didn't research it. Yes, it falls out. Now, maybe some of you already shave down there and will be happy about this. For the rest of us it's weird. Not as weird as being bald up top, but still weird. Hair falls out from the rest of your body, too. You'll have the smoothest skin for a while and not have to shave your legs. See? Upside. Chemo nose (the constant running) is caused by the fact that your nose hairs fall out, and so your nose is irritated all the time. When they grow back—voilà—no more runny nose.

GETTING WIGGY AND
THE ART OF SCARF TYING

I could write a whole book on what it feels like and how to handle being bald. Or, I could sum it up with this:

IT SUCKS

There isn't a font big enough to describe accurately how much it sucks. I'm not saying this to scare you.

I'm telling you this so you know how much time is spent in support groups and coffee shops and doctors' offices discussing how very much this affects women. You're already programmed to obsess over this. You've suffered through bad hair days, terrible haircuts, the works. You know how your hair can affect your mood. Guess what? Having no hair affects you even more.

Okay, so now that you know the truth, let's get to the nitty-gritty. How do you deal with it? Most cancer centers around the country have a few free wigs and hats for patients. You can go to your local chapter and see what they've got. There's also a catalog in every oncologist's office with a selection of hats and scarves you can order. The first time you flip through this catalog you will most likely still have a full head of hair, and you will giggle and remark about how absurd some of the items look. Some time later, bald as a cue ball, you will flip through that same catalog and consider whether that crocheted hat with the stick-on bangs might look better on you in white or black. Funny how the search for the perfect accessory moves quickly from which handbag—to which bag of hair. There are also many wig shops around the country. Just check the yellow pages, ask in your oncologist's office, the local American Cancer Society chapter, and so on. There are many resources for wigs, both synthetic and human hair.

Wigs have two different ways of attaching. Most have an elastic band built right in. The custom ones have a kind of skullcap that you use wig tape to stick on. And here's what you're now going to worry about: You'll get out of your car, wig askew, and run into an acquaintance in the parking lot who will be trying not to stare. A sitcom-worthy moment.

I promise you this will not happen. Neither one of these types of attachments will let the wig fly off your head. Today's wigs fit extremely well, and, on your bald head, you will feel it if it moves even slightly out of place.

There are some nice synthetic wigs that look quite real and are super easy to care for. For synthetic wigs you need: (1) a wide-tooth comb; (2) dish soap. To style a synthetic-hair wig you have to—do *nothing*! Seriously, how cool is that? You literally wash it out with a little dish soap and water in the sink and hang it up to dry. I hung mine on the faucet knob in the shower. When it's dry you comb it with a wide-tooth comb and voilà—perfect every time. If you have problem hair in real life, you may actually like this part. Okay, only for a minute, but it's a good minute. A friend of mine told me that after her own hair grew back and she stopped wearing her wig, a friend said, "You should really go back to wearing your hair the other way. It looked much better." She had to break the news to her that it was a wig.

One "friend" of mine told me I was lucky—yes, lucky—to have to wear a wig because it's so much easier than styling your own hair: It must save me so much time in the morning. Uh-huh. So lucky. That's just how I felt every morning when I slapped that synthetic-hair hat on my bald head. Oh, thank goodness I have all this extra time to get ready to go dancing! Yes, people say the darnedest things.

The place on your head that a wig looks the most artificial is right along your "hairline." Especially at the top of your forehead and around your ears. It's where your own hairline normally has little baby hairs that soften the edges. Wigs don't do that, even the really expensive ones. They can't because of the way the hair is sewn into the structure. I asked Kurt, my wig guy (who would have thought I'd have a wig guy?), why the wigs in the movies look so much more natural, and he told me that in the movies they use a piece that comes down over the forehead, and then they cover that with makeup to create a more realistic hairline. It takes hours, and if you saw it in real life, it wouldn't look as real as you think. Wigs with bangs are better at camouflaging this area, but there are always going to be areas that are not quite perfect.

So, it's never going to look like real hair—to you. But for most people it will. It will look so real that people who know your situation may talk about it, which is just plain uncomfortable. Once a fellow patient at the cancer center came up to me in the waiting room and said, "I've been watching you all these weeks, and I just can't believe you haven't lost your hair yet. You're so lucky." I was happy to inform her I was in the same boat as she—totally bald but with a good wig.

The worst part is when somebody wants to pat you on the head. I'm not sure why people feel the need to do this, ever, but occasionally this happens. They will not know just from patting you that something is amiss, but I will tell you it is one of the strangest feelings ever. It is kind of like when someone goes to take your glasses off your face, and you want to pull back and say, *Do not touch!* Excuse yourself from obsessing. We all do it at this point.

TOP 5 TIPS FOR WIG WEARERS

1. Try on a bunch of wig styles and colors. You may find that, with your new situation, something different than you're used to actually works best. And while you're at it, there's nothing wrong with having a little fun and trying something you've always wondered about.

2. You can, and maybe should, take your wig to your regular hair stylist and ask her to trim it to look more appropriate for you. Wear it on your head for this. Don't bring in the Styrofoam wig stand and expect her to cut it while you go grocery shopping. Having it done is a little like cutting the hair on your doll when you were six, though. Remember, it doesn't grow back, so less is more. My stylist cried when I came in, but she had the decency to run in the back first. If you've had a long relationship with your stylist, expect some sort of reaction, because it's really personal to them.

3. If you have a real-hair wig, the best way to style it is while it's on your head. Wash it first in the sink with some diluted shampoo. Then do the same thing

with conditioner, and then plop it on your head after you squeeze some of the water out. This does not feel good. In fact, it's kind of like pulling on a pair of wet jeans. Also, you can't get the same kind of tension with a hairbrush as you do with your own hair, because the wig's not on that tight. But blow-drying it and styling it on your head is still the best way to get it to look more or less right.

4. You don't have to wash a wig as often as you wash your own hair because there are no hair follicles, and it doesn't get as dirty as fast. There you go—another small blessing. Remember, I told you to appreciate them where you can!

5. Your doctor can write you a wig prescription. Yes, you can get a little money from your insurance for a rug. It won't cover the price of the more expensive ones, but it will help a little. Hmmm . . . wonder if we can get extras for husbands?

My favorite thing when I was switching wigs all the time was when my daughter's friend kept telling me how much she liked my new haircuts. She didn't see me all that much, so one day it would be long and reddish with bangs. Then it would be my own—dark, wavy, shoulder length. Then the next time, short and sassy. Finally, after a few months, my daughter mentioned that I had breast cancer, and only then did the lightbulb go on. It had just never occurred to her, but each time she commented I had this urge to tell her.

That urge is something that comes and goes throughout the whole process. Especially when people comment on your hairstyle. Even when it's growing out and you get compliments on how cute your short hair looks from people who don't know, you may feel impelled to say, "Thanks. I went to Chemo Cuts."

GROWING BACK—THE HAIR, I MEAN

First there's the tiniest bit of stubble on your scalp. For many of us, all manner of rejoicing starts in that moment. I figured that was it, right? I'd read all the books, so I knew it could come in differently than before, etc. But what *really* happens is that a little bit of stubble grows from the follicles that were there the whole time—the 1 percent or whatever that never fell out—that you had to shave down. That hair starts to grow. Just for a little while. Just long enough for you to feel it, know you aren't going to shave it because *it's growing back, yippee*!!!! And then . . . nothing. For a few weeks I checked daily. Okay, hourly, but that's not important. It stops. And then one day you become aware that there is this fuzz around your scalp. Yes, fuzz. I've asked around, and everyone says the same thing. And it's colorless. The hair grows back colorless. Not white or gray but actually colorless. Now that stubble is still there, too, which is kind of weird, but who cares, right? It's *growing back*! And now you wait.

You will most likely get some scalp sensitivity during this time. Oh, by the way, whenever you read "sensitivity" in a book about cancer and treatment, insert "a little pain" instead. In this case it's not bad at all, but there may be some pain when you touch those hairs. Kind of like when you get an ingrown hair from shaving. And you can get some little pimple-like sore spots.

Okay, so now your head is covered in this fuzz, and then all of a sudden a few of them start to turn toward their natural color. Not all the hairs, but some. The longer they are, the more color you start to see. It takes weeks, but it happens. My husband and I liked the way it felt. Kind of like running your hand over a really short buzz cut, only there aren't as many hairs. Don't misunderstand: At this point you are still effectively bald, but it's like those first buds in March. Spring is coming!

My hair started growing from the sides and back first. This was more than a little disturbing. I had a fringe of hair around my ears but the top was still shiny bald. Not exactly what I had in mind. Looking like a monk was not sexy. After a couple of weeks, it started to fill in very slowly at the top. Still patchy and colorless, but at least it was growing. By the time it starts to grow in all over your head, you will notice it's growing back in other parts of your body as well. In my case, in the same weird pattern. Pubic hair started growing back on the fringes, not right in the middle. It's male-pattern baldness in reverse. The pubic hair thing really got to me. It just looked so darn strange down there. Maybe that's just me. Unfortunately this also means you have to start shaving your legs again, and that smoothness all over your skin starts to disappear as the rest of your body starts to grow hair again. Oh well, it's still worth it. Oddly, the hair under my right arm (surgery side) took months longer to start to reappear. The trauma of surgery seems to affect the growth there.

When those little colorless hairs get to be about half an inch long, and the color starts to come in, the hairs now look like porcupine quills, with white on the ends and color beneath. I kept wearing wigs for a little while, but this is when I started to feel really comfortable wearing scarves. Perhaps it's just that by the end of nine months I was more comfortable being recognized as Cancer Girl. Also, that tiny bit of hair around your hairline seems to make a huge difference. It just looks a lot more "normal" (notice the quotes). I think the biggest change for me, though, was that I just got sick of wearing a hair hat.

All the effort to look a certain way got to me eventually. I started to feel like I was doing it for everyone on the outside, and so I transitioned to scarves. And then the week I finished radiation, I had my coming-out party. I went to my stylist and had a little color wash put in so it wasn't so colorless, and I stopped wearing any covering and lived with the hair I had. People still stared. I mean, it still didn't look like a purposeful hairstyle or anything, but I just couldn't care anymore. I just felt it was time. And it was one less thing to worry about.

Eyelashes grow back differently than the rest of your hair. It's as if one day you have none, and then the next day you have a whole line. It's wonderful. They may be just stubs, but those stubs do more to make you look normal than anything that's happened in a long time. Of course then you realize that they stay short for *sooo* long!

TOP 5 TIPS WHEN YOUR HAIR STARTS GROWING BACK—YAY!

1. Keep using the scalp shampoo from Aveda with the exfoliating properties, because it seems to cut down on many of the scalp issues I'd heard about, including dry itchy scalp (mine still itched, but not as bad as some), ingrown hairs, and other lumps and bumps. And it smells good and foams up, which is oddly comforting. I knew there was no actual hair being washed up there, but I still preferred cleaning the area with something that acted and smelled like shampoo. I haven't checked with the Aveda company, but I'm guessing this was part of their thinking in the design of the product, which is really intended for balding men.

2. Use an electric razor on any part of your body that is slightly numb. Otherwise you run the risk of cutting yourself, and that could lead to lymphedema.

3. Try using mascara that has the word *lengthening* on it. They often come with a primer or base coat, and if you get one with fibers or little "beauty tubes," they act like little extensions for your sad

little stubs. Also, the over-the-counter growth mascara may help. Some of my friends said they thought it did.

4. Check with your local American Cancer Society chapter for makeup sessions. They occasionally run makeup seminars for cancer patients to teach them how to apply makeup that makes your face look brighter and gives the appearance of having eyelashes and eyebrows.

5. Check with your local health-food store for vitamins with biotin. The bottles usually say "for hair and nails" on them, and some of my friends swear they worked.

SCARVES AND HATS

There are a whole slew of options. That's the good news. The bad news is that people will stare. They just can't help themselves. You cannot hide your diagnosis in a scarf or hat. More power to you if you just don't care. Most kids, it seems, prefer that Mom walk around in a wig. It's easier to imagine a healthy you if there's hair. However, if you're a scarf girl (and I was, for part of the time), here's my scarf advice.

TOP 5 TIPS FOR WEARING
SCARVES AND HATS

1. A scarf on a totally bald head does not look like Rhoda, who was clearly making a choice. The reason people tie all sorts of extra stuff around the top and front of the scarf is that when you put it on and have no hair under it, the top is just way too flat. Hair lifts up at the hairline. A scarf over skin does not and seems to accentuate the baldness under it. That's why scarves have all those twisty knots; they distract from the total smoothness underneath.

2. Local cancer centers often have scarf-tying lessons and a whole host of helpful hints, Web links, and tips.

3. Baseball hats do not cover the area around your ears or the back of your neck, so they can accentuate the baldness factor.

4. Having a long scarf trailing down your neck can feel kind of like long hair, so it's nice to have that weight and swing back there.

5. Scarves look better with earrings, too! My husband kept hoping I'd take my wig off in public.

Something about the shock value of it appealed to him, I guess. I just kept envisioning horror movies where the kids run screaming from the monster. In actuality I did have moments where I pulled my hat or wig off in the car to be more comfortable. I tried not to look at the other drivers. One night, though, I gave my husband a present. We went out to dinner to celebrate a work thing for him, and it was just the two of us. I started having a hot flash and whipped off my wig in the middle of the restaurant. He was floored—and loved it. The waitress pretended not to be shocked, and I sat there for the rest of dinner, naked head. Very liberating, but also kind of like the dream where you realize you've gone to school without your clothes on.

My kids had varying reactions to my being bald. In the very beginning they didn't even want to see me in a scarf. It just said "cancer" and "scary" in big shiny white letters. As time wore on, and there were hats and various wigs and scarves, they got used to it. At one point my daughter, who said very little to me about my treatment during this whole process, but was a real trouper and helped hugely, said, "Mom, you don't have to wear a wig or hat for me. You should be comfortable." Nearly brought me to tears.

However, leaving wigs lying around the house was never popular. Sometimes I would just pull it off wherever I was at home to be more comfortable and then forget to put it back on. My daughter, as cool as she was during the whole bald thing, did not appreciate finding a strange "animal" on the kitchen counter next to a plate of cut-up fruit. Can't imagine why not!

MORE HAIR

Six months after the end of chemo, I finally had hair. Actual hair. I had it colored several times and it didn't fall out, so I tell everyone that as soon as your doctor says it's okay to color it, go right ahead. My stylist started with a color wash instead of the usual heavy-duty dye, and just having it kind of back to my normal color was a huge feeling of relief. There's a great deal of talk online about when you should color it, but as long as your skin isn't too sensitive and you use a gentle product, you should be okay.

Everyone says your hair grows back curly. My personal experience is that after that first bit of weird, thin chemo hair gets cut off, what came in was my hair, only supercurly. However, if you haven't ever had short hair, or it's been a while, you may not know what your hair texture is when it's supershort. Remember, you are literally starting from scratch. I swore once my hair came in I would never complain about having bad-hair days again but—yikes! Curls, curls everywhere, and complain I did (and still do a little).

Aside from looking like I'd spent the day at the beauty parlor having my hair set the way my grandma did thirty years ago, I felt like this hair I was sporting was leaving a false impression. For women, having short hair seems to imply something. Whether it's that you're "funky," "sporty," "self-confident" (all adjectives that came up in discussion with friends about this issue), whatever, it does leave an impression. I found it a little disturbing. Not as much as being bald—I mean that's *really* disturbing—but still, something didn't sit quite right. During this time of the very short hair, we moved to Santa Barbara, California. It was summer, and I was actually quite enjoying the freedom of not having my usual heavy long locks, but something was bugging me, and I finally figured out what it was. It felt like people's first impressions of me were going to be compromised. I felt as though I needed a sign that said, "This is not how I look."

Moving and meeting new people put it in perspective for me, because my friends and family knew this was not my chosen look, but new people couldn't know. They would assume I was one of those adjectives: "sporty," "strong," "cool," "funky," and so on. I am, in fact, neither funky nor sporty and, during this time, not self-confident either. I talked this out with my husband. He said he feels the same way about looking in the mirror as he ages; the reflection doesn't match the persona. So I guess many people feel that way, but like a lot of things after cancer, it's magnified.

For many women in the CSC—Cancer Sucks Club—I think the biggest problem with supershort hair (not to mention the one boob or fewer, lest we forget) is not feeling feminine. I am sure if you started with short hair, this does not have as big an impact at this stage, but for those of us who started with some length, it doesn't matter how many people say you look beautiful or cute or whatever, it still is hard not to feel stripped of femininity during this time.

Of course some people say all the right things. They tell you that your face is so striking that you can really carry off the short look. Nobody's going to tell you that you look bad with your new hair, though, unless you have really mean friends.

My kids were able to talk to me about this issue.

They told me how strange it was to see me drive up to get them, because they kept expecting the woman in the car to have long dark hair. Instead it was just me.

About this time, I met a new friend in my support group. She had been through chemotherapy more recently than I. We talked about the hair situation often. She told me how hard it was for her to deal with, and I reassured her that I knew precisely what she was going through. She said, "But you look so great with short hair! It suits your face." I told her thanks, but really, I knew what she was feeling. I could tell she thought I was just being nice, so I decided to put on my Andrea wig, the one made with my own hair, and show her just how much I understood what she was going through. I hadn't worn it in a few months, and I'd grown accustomed to seeing myself with short hair.

We stood in my bathroom. She whipped off her wig, and we examined her head and new growth. Then I got mine out of the box. As soon as I put it on, she said, "Ohhh." Softly. Suddenly she could see part of the "me" I had lost. When I looked in the mirror, I felt an intense feeling of recognition. Aha! That's what I remembered. In fact, it was so much more powerful than when I had worn it all those times before, because for the first time in a very long time, my face looked healthy beneath the hair.

It was an emotional moment for both of us. Until I saw the gardeners looking in my bathroom window. We burst out laughing. I swear my gardener hasn't been able to look me in the eye since. I'm thinking it was worse than seeing me naked. Well, maybe not.

I started looking around at all the women I saw with really short hair, wondering how many of them had recently finished treatment. How many of those confident-looking women had endured what I had just gone through? How many were walking around with a weighty prosthesis dragging on their chests or were sporting the same slice of scar I have?

I wish I could tell you when you will start to recognize yourself in the mirror. Maybe it depends on how short your hair was to begin with. After a year I was still waiting. I *can* tell you that you look better than you think you do. *You are not objective.* Neither is your family. The truth is, your family sees you both looking more beautiful and less like yourself than you do. It's a weird dichotomy. They see the real you and don't really care about your hair, so they see the pretty where you can't. On the other hand, just like you, given a choice they'd probably prefer the hair you used to have, so don't ask them to choose. Or tell you which is better. Or when it's time to say goodbye to the wig. As I said to a friend the other day, it's not like a pair of shoes that wears through or goes out of style. How your family sees you right now is tied up in a million different feelings, so don't ask them what you should do about your hair. You'll hate every answer they give you.

TOP 5 TIPS FOR
THE GROWING-OUT STAGE

1. Do not air-dry your hair—curls get curlier.

2. Buy a tiny flatiron and use it—with any kind of protectant cream first—as soon as you have enough hair with color in it to fit between the little bars. But don't overdo it; you don't want to burn the hair you have.

3. Color your hair as soon as your oncologist says you can. There's a lot of chatter about this on the Web, but the only one to listen to is your oncologist. Remember: You need to trust her, above and beyond the advice of your well-meaning friends. I started at my salon with just a little nonpermanent wash and as my hair grew, went on to the hard stuff. It made a big difference to me to at least see my "natural" color. And, no, it did not fall out!

---

4. Don't worry about the stares. You're inevitably going to get them, because it's not quite normal-looking yet.

5. Once you come out, you can't go back. Well, it's tricky anyway. After the first time I went without, that was it for me. I figured once I was out, I was out and proud. My friend did it a little at a time. She would occasionally go out without her wig, then put it back on. I kept thinking it would be weirder for someone to see her with short funky hair one day and long the next than just thinking she'd gotten a really cool haircut.

How long does it take? I'm not going to lie. It takes a year and a half before it's long enough for even a mini-ponytail. My friend's daughter called it a "phonytail." By the time you get to that stage, you'll be so happy with it you won't care that there are a million bobby pins holding it back. Just the idea that you can play with it enough to actually work with it is a huge relief. This is the stage you can start to ask your stylist about extensions.

7

Radiation

I'm calling this the KFC phase: Kentucky Fried Chicken. Or Kindle (not the e-reader) Fry Char. Okay, it's really not that bad for most people, but you will get crispy, and not in that teenager-sunburned-at-the-beach-wearing-coconut-oil kind of way. More in the your-mother-told-you-to-wear-sunscreen-but-you-forgot-and-spent-the-day-on-a-boat kind of way. I had my radiation treatments after surgery and chemotherapy, but you may have them first.

There is actually a little preparation the doctors put you through before they start radiation, and nobody told me exactly what it would entail. Or maybe they did, but I was so hopped up on steroids and chemo drugs that it didn't sink in. Here's a summary, in case you, too, have chemo-induced brain fog:

PLANNING AND PLOTTING

First come the planning sessions, where they basically plot a graph on you and tattoo you—ouch! The tattoos are marks that, later on, will help the technicians line up the radiation machine. The idea is to identify exactly where to aim the beam so that it destroys all the cancer cells and as few healthy cells as possible. To figure it out they put you into a CT scanner, which lets them map your body. That first day you start out feeling like a drawing pad, because they really mark you up with ink and Sharpie pens.

Then they take the key points and use a needle to tattoo them. For those of us who are uncool enough to still be ink-free at this point, here's a heads-up: Getting a tattoo stings. It's a needle stick through an ink spot, and some hurt more than others. The tattoos themselves are just tiny bluish dots. They're barely visible, but they are permanent. Nobody told me that. It's as though they think you won't care because of all the other stuff you're going through. I'm sorry, but I care about any permanent mark that's being made on my body. Especially the ones I didn't choose. Whether it's a scar or a tiny blue dot. They really are teeny, tiny dots, but, hey, I didn't put them there! I was hoping for a little heart or something. Maybe a unicorn, but you only get dots. Thereafter, every time you go for treatment, they use those tattoos as guides to line up the field of treatment and pinpoint the radiation.

The tattooing session can also be painful because they have to put you in whatever position they're going to have to repeat during the radiation, so make sure you stretch before and after. The tattooing techs may not be the same as those who will actually perform the radiation; these are just people who make the blueprints—on you.

TOP 5 TIPS FOR THE FIRST RADIATION APPOINTMENT

1. Wash off the marker ink as soon as you can, because otherwise you can get a shadow where they drew on you, and it takes forever to wear off.

2. Stretch before you go, especially the area around your surgery, and take pain medication about an hour beforehand if you're postsurgical, because you may have to hold an awkward position during the initial setting-up process, and it can hurt. Even something as basic as acetaminophen helps.

---

3. Be prepared for multiple tiny but ouchy pinpricks. The number of spots you'll get depends on how many sites they have to radiate.

4. Wear loose clothing, and try to leave your modesty at the door, because you're going to have to bare your chest.

5. Do not make tattoo jokes to the technicians. They don't think it's funny.

I'm not going to lie: I whined a lot during this session. I'm not sure why. Was it because I'd already been through so much and I'd just about had it? Was it because I was still in pain and recovering from surgery and chemo? I don't know, but I've talked to lots of people, and everyone seems to have been surprised by this process. I wasn't the only whiner. I'm guessing it has something to do with the lack of a decent warning. I think most radiation oncologists kind of bypass an information session on the prep portion of radiation. Personally I hate surprises unless they come in a velvet box, so I'm giving you a heads-up. It's not horrible, but the tattoos do hurt, and the session can be uncomfortable.

PREHEAT

On radiation days (five days a week for nearly seven weeks), you change into a gown and sit in a waiting room with the other radiation patients. You can always ask someone for a warm blanket to wrap around your shoulders if you need one. Then your techs call you back to your machine. You'll probably be in the same room every time. The techs may switch in and out, but, of the two or three assigned to you, there is always one familiar face every day.

I was kind of shocked when I went the first time, because there were men in the waiting room in their drawstring pajama bottoms. I don't know why it never occurred to me that radiation centers deal with all kinds of cancers, but I just never thought about it. And then there they were, all looking rather sad and vulnerable. So just letting you know—you're going to see it all here at the Cancer Club. And let me tell you— sometimes the view is not pretty. However, there's a sense of community in all these waiting rooms. You all belong to the same club now. Different chapters, but still the same club.

I found that the conversations rarely crossed the gender gap. Too up-close and personal, is my guess. If you're interested, though, it's easy to strike up conversations in the waiting rooms, because you see the same faces every day. Everyone I talked to found their radiation experiences to be the most convivial of all the treatments. The techs, nurses, and patients all seem more willing to share than in the other wings. I think it's because, for the most part, people feel pretty well when they undergo radiation. They may be a little crispy by the end, but they're still cheerful.

BAKE

What's radiation like? The daily experience is not that bad. This is how it works: Now that you have the tattoos, all they have to do is connect the dots. Literally. After you check in and change into your gown, a lovely person calls you into the radiation room. You have to walk through a door with one of those nuclear signs on it. You know—the kind with the three triangles. You untie your gown and lie down on a narrow table. The machine is behind the table, and after you lie down, the tech moves the table with a remote control so it slides back toward the machine. Then they manipulate you so you are in position for the beams. They line up your dots in the beam field so they radiate only where they're supposed to. Everyone will try very hard to make you feel comfortable, but you're probably not. They ask you to relax, and then they manipulate your body by using the sheet you're lying on; they pull it and roll you just a little at a time until you're in the right position. The table moves up and down and side to side until it's exactly right. Then a large round piece of equipment moves around you into position. During all this time, one tech is most likely drawing on you with a Sharpie or washable pen. Just think of yourself as a specimen on the slide of a microscope. When everything is all lined up, the techs leave the room. The machine clicks and then buzzes, and usually, a sign that says "Beam On" lights up. Depending on your position, you may or may not be able to see it. Then the door opens, and they come back and move the table to the next position.

There's no pain from the radiation itself. You may have muscle pain later from being in an awkward position, but the beam causes no sensation at all. Really! My arm and hand went numb from how I was positioned, but that's about it.

The truth is, though, you are going to have some skin side effects. I was humming along throughout the whole process, feeling quite smug. Every day they would tell me how great my skin looked, and I thought I had it beat. I had come up with the magic potion and routine, and was going to share it in this book and save so many people from suffering. It didn't quite work out according to plan. Yes, my advice on aloe and calendula cream is real and helpful and prevents a lot of pain and burning. My skin was just mildly pink all the way to the end of my seven-week cycle. My radiation oncologist was thrilled. Everyone asked me my secret, which I happily shared. I was told that the effects don't peak until a week to nine days after the end of treatment, so I kept up with all my lotions and potions. And then right on schedule, things started to happen. Not nice things. The skin under my arm stared to blister and turn red. Actually, it was more like mahogany. I continued my routine, but nothing could stop what was going on. The whole area in and around my armpit blistered and peeled. In my case, I was a little lucky that part of that area was still numb from the surgery, but not enough. *Ouch!*

I've talked to many women who had radiation who suffered less than I did. And many who suffered more. The ones who suffered less, to a one, did not have their armpits radiated. So if your fate is to have your armpits radiated, raise your hand and don't put it down for seven weeks. I was really worried about the skin on my chest, because I had the most treatment there, with a bolus (an extra layer of what looks like bubble wrap that they lay on you to moderate the amount of radiation on certain areas) as well, but that never got as bad as under my arm. That area just got pink and sensitive. When I say "just," I am not for one minute diminishing its impact on my life, but it just wasn't as bad as the other part of me.

One weird thing to notice is how perfect the line is between radiated skin and nonradiated skin. I thought it was just remarkable that you could see a real rectangle where the beam hit. Hey, you have to find something to amuse yourself, right? You may also find that you have some pink or itchy dry skin on your back. I didn't get this, but I know several women who did. It depends on the angle of radiation.

The good news is that blistering, peeling, oozing sensitive skin does heal. It really does peak at around nine days, and then you can see a noticeable decline in new areas of pain and blistering. Unfortunately this does not mean that the pain starts to go away on day ten; it just means that nothing new happens, and this is an improvement in itself. Very quickly, though, the pain starts to decrease and new skin forms. And then you can spend your days peeling at that dry, cracked skin until it's all gone. Lovely. I do recommend wearing loose cotton shirts to bed to protect your sheets from all the goop. I won't define "goop" for you—you get the idea.

Skin problems are only one of the side effects of radiation. I read all the literature and saw the word "fatigue" and thought I knew what that meant. I mean, after surgery and chemotherapy, I had seen that word fifty times already. I knew that it meant a two p.m. nap for me every day. Right? Oh *sooo* wrong! The side effects of radiation are real. The profound fatigue is real. In my case I started radiation seven months after diagnosis. This, following multiple tests, surgery, and chemotherapy. I was also on the oral medication lapatinib. The fatigue I felt started around the third week of radiation. It felt different from the fatigue during chemotherapy; that was more like hitting a wall at a certain point in the day. Radiation fatigue is more like a daily slog. Every morning I woke up tired and stayed that way. Some days I was more functional than others, but it was always a struggle to get even the most minor things done. I felt like I could have slept from morning to—the next morning, and it still wouldn't have been enough. It was like wearing a lead suit every day, all day. I could do literally one thing a day, and that was it.

I know a number of women who went through radiation and still held full-time jobs. It's definitely possible. I only hope none of them are pilots, surgeons, or crane operators, because some days even getting to the hospital was all I could do. If you are one of those people who can just pop in for radiation, then do a full day's work and take care of your kids, my hat goes off to you. I dragged myself around for those last weeks, just counting the days.

I actually had one of the worst moments of my treatment after the first week of radiation. I woke up, and after talking in bed with my husband for a while and feeling relatively normal, I got up and looked in the mirror and totally fell apart. There, in the bathroom in the morning light, I saw a pale, bald, one-breasted, old-looking woman with a huge scar. Fingers red with peeling fingernails, no eyelashes and ink marks from the radiation all up and down her arm and chest. Truly a horrific sight. I just lost it. I felt so ugly. I cried and cried. Then my husband came in and asked what was wrong, and when I told him, he just looked at me and said, "You are not ugly, and this is temporary. All the things you see are temporary." It took a few minutes for me to calm down, but once I did I realized he was right, and it helped. I put on my wig and a smile and went down for breakfast feeling just a little brighter. One week down—only six more to go! There are days when you will feel ugly and overwhelmed. It helps to remember that it is all temporary. Your body will recover. Your hair will grow back. The pain, fatigue, nausea, and other side effects will subside. The skin burns will heal, and there will be a day in the not-too-distant future when you will look in the mirror and see a familiar sight. I promise.

THE AFTERBURN

They tell you that your skin continues to suffer from the effects of radiation for a week or two after you finish. As I mentioned, they told me the effects would peak at about ten days after the last treatment. So I waited and watched. I continued to apply all the ointments and treatments I've listed for you below. I watched the skin go from light pink to cranberry and then to an almost burgundy color. I watched the bubbles form. I did the saline soak and tried to stem the tide of pain and peeling. No such luck. I was powerless and at the mercy of my skin.

It peeled and peeled again. Keep in mind that radiation is not like a sunburn, which only affects the top layer of skin. Radiation goes deeper, so when the first layer of skin bubbles and peels away, it reveals a new layer that needs to peel away as well. All you can do is keep applying the saline soak and calendula creams. The worst areas are the ones where your skin rubs up against itself, like in your armpit. *Ouch!*

TOP 5 TIPS FOR PROTECTING YOUR SKIN DURING RADIATION

1. Ask them to put a warm blanket under you on the table. Boy, do I love warm blankets!

2. If they have to use a bolus, ask them to lay it on your legs first to warm it up. Otherwise they plop it on your skin, and it's freezing!

3. Apparently the worst reactions to radiation occur when your skin rubs against itself. The only way to prevent this from happening to you is to keep your arm raised as much as possible. I'm not kidding! If I could do it all again—and I pray nightly that I never, ever have to do any of this again—I would walk around with my hand on my hip and seriously do everything I could to avoid having anything rub against any part of radiated skin. Let me tell you, it would be worth it if you could save yourself from the pain of the burning, cracking, peeling skin.

4. Bring 100 percent aloe gel with you every day and apply it while you are getting dressed again. Following every treatment, apply calendula cream (or whatever cream your doctor recommends) three

times a day. Basically, apply all the right creams, as much as you can.

5. I also used a saline wash (a half teaspoon of salt in a bowl of lukewarm distilled water, applied with a clean lint-free cloth) once a day as close to the treatment as possible. Most doctors recommend it for when the skin gets really red, but I started right away. You can also apply cornstarch to the skin; it's very soothing. After your final treatment, if you blister and peel, try using A+D ointment and Bag Balm along with the other products. Anything that's safe on burns is okay to use. I even used Desitin to keep the chafing to a minimum. I smelled like a baby for a week, and basically wore the same two shirts over and over, because they were the only things that didn't touch the sensitive areas on my body.

The good news is that the effects of radiation wear off very quickly, and you can move on to bigger and better things.

8

How "Normal" Is the New Normal?

This is one of the hardest things about the whole ordeal: How do you define "normal" when your whole world has turned upside down? Is it when you feel well enough to go to a dinner party, and you look great in your new wig, but during dessert you have to run to the bathroom and rip it off because you're having a hot flash? Or is it when you figure out how to wear your cotton puff (code for "fake boob") in a way that matches your other breast so nobody can tell? Is it when you actually think you may want to have sex with your partner, but then when you start, all you can think of is your bald head (even though he says he doesn't care)? People talk about the "new normal." I found that for me and many others, all that means is that every day is a new day. Every day your body feels different. Every day you will feel different. Some days are good days, and on those days you may want to spend a few hours not feeling like a cancer patient, just doing something normal. Even though your blood counts may be low or you may not be looking great. Then, when you're about to start, or when you suggest doing something that you used to do, people say, "You can't do that!" As in, you can't go to the movies—you have cancer. You can't go shopping at the mall—you have cancer! You cannot possibly drive yourself to the grocery store—*you have cancer*! Even being able to do those little things can go a long way toward helping you feel normal.

Some days all you want to do is forget, and it seems as if all people do is remind you. And most of them are people you love and who love you. Your family may be the worst offenders. If you're lucky (like me), all they want to do is protect you and keep you safe and well. But sometimes, no matter how well meaning they are, they go too far. They might suggest you ignore what the doctor says in favor of some conventional wisdom. They may want you to see some other doctor they heard was "the one." They may call and tell you they just heard about someone who received some new treatment somewhere. The fact is that only you and your doctors have the information and tools to determine what you can and cannot do. What is a risk and what is not. Listen to your doctors and your own body. Tune out the others. You will survive this experience happier and healthier if you can learn to say, "Thank you. I know you mean well, but I've discussed this with my doctor and it's okay."

Part of the new normal is feeling out of control. One day you're an adult, pretty much in charge of your own life and body; and the next day you are at the mercy of a disease, its treatment, and the medical community. Your very own body has turned against you. To recapture some measure of control, you may find you do unusual things. You may become obsessed by an article of clothing, or a song, or the way a meal is prepared. You may look in the mirror fifty times a day or avoid mirrors altogether. You may all of a sudden become germophobic or agoraphobic. You get the idea. Is this "normal"? When "normal" is being stuck by a needle every week and hooked up to poison, then all bets are off. The trick is not to be self-destructive. Staying home in your pj's watching *Say Yes to the Dress* instead of going to a PTA meeting—okay. Avoiding treatment—not okay. Going to the mall because your doc says you're well enough—okay. Going on an Antarctic trek without telling anyone—not okay.

You will find there are scads of people out there with incredibly generous spirits. Some will surprise you with their kindnesses. One neighbor whom I rarely talked to would occasionally drop bags of groceries at my door, completely unannounced. One lovely woman changed her work schedule without telling me (I heard it from another friend), just in case I needed a ride to chemo. Friends of friends offered meals, rides, company, support.

Then there are the "finers." The people who treat you like everything's fine. Let's assume that more than half of them just don't know what else to do. Maybe they are very private people themselves, and so they don't want to say anything, because they think you wouldn't want them to. Or they don't know how to say what they feel, don't know what to do, so they do nothing. Forgive them. Or help them find the words or actions that you need. Talk about what you're going through openly, if that's what makes you feel comfortable, or ask them to cook a meal or pick up your kids because you're too tired. It's easy to misinterpret nonaction as noncaring.

I thought I was good friends with one of my neighbors. Our children were very close, and we'd spent many happy occasions and holiday parties together. We'd gone out for walks and dinners and talked quite a bit on the phone. She was one of the first people I told. She is a warm and helpful person, and I fully expected her to show up with meals and flowers and laughs every so often. Instead we had very little contact. I didn't understand it at all. Then one day I saw her when we were both getting into our cars, and we started talking. She burst into tears and apologized for not being around, but she really didn't know what to do. She said she was just overcome by what I was going through and didn't know how to help or what to say. What seemed so obvious to me—a phone call, a visit, a batch of brownies—was beyond her. Something so small seemed perfect to me but not enough for her, and so she was frozen. Our talk helped her through it, and after that she was wonderful.

Another friend was so struck by what had happened to me that the only way she could deal with it was to become obsessed with her own health. As you can imagine, this wasn't helpful to me in the least, but that was how she could cope.

Then there are the people who are just plain inappropriate. I had one (and only one, thank goodness) experience with a woman who kept calling me while I was still in treatment. I had been at a Super Bowl party, apparently not looking like death warmed over (I won't tell you how long it took me to create that illusion), and a few weeks later she called to ask me to meet with her about a charity event. I told her I couldn't do it that week. She called once a week for a month, wanting to get together. Keep in mind, by now I'm having radiation. I kept saying no. When she refused to give up, I finally e-mailed her and said, "As I'm sure you know, I'm in treatment right now, and as I'm sure you've discovered by my inability to meet with you, my days are kind of crazy. I'm reserving what little energy I have for my family and healing." She wrote back that she was sorry to keep pestering me, but since she had seen me out and about she "assumed I was feeling better." Feeling better? *Feeling better?* Are you kidding me? I'm in the middle of cancer treatment, and she thinks she knows how I feel because I had a wig and makeup on one day? "Feeling better" is a trick phrase. I didn't have the flu, I had cancer.

One woman told me that her adult daughter came to stay with her during chemo, ostensibly to help, but somehow she always ended up on the couch watching TV while her mother was doing laundry, cooking, and cleaning. It was hard for her to remind her daughter that she was the patient and needed to be waited on a little. Not the other way around. This reversal of roles can be very challenging. For husbands, too. However, you have to do what it takes to take care of yourself. This is a time to put yourself first and ask for help when you need it. You really will not be able to go through treatment and still do everything you're used to doing. It just doesn't work that way. And most of your friends will step up, I promise.

TOP 5 TIPS FOR DEALING WITH PEOPLE

1. Don't be afraid to tell people you are not up for something if you feel you're not. Don't be afraid to leave early. Try not to bite someone's head off when they assume you're fine because you look well. People who haven't gone through this have no idea how much effort it takes to look even remotely human.

2. Do not put on a show unless it makes you feel better. It is not your responsibility to make other people feel more comfortable around you. This is a topic discussed many times in support groups (more about them later; they can be incredibly helpful). We feel responsible for making sure everyone

else is okay with the fact that we're sick. Looking backward—that's backward!

3. Save what little energy you have for the things that you have to do or that make you feel better. For crying out loud, just getting to treatment every day and getting dressed can be draining enough some days. If you also have to work and/or take care of kids, that's all anyone should have to handle.

4. You have my permission, and the permission of everyone in my support group, to lash out appropriately at anyone who makes you feel uncomfortable. I know lots of women whose children, coworkers, spouses, stepmothers, etc., said something along the lines of "Enough already." As in, enough talk about how tired, bald, uncomfortable, scared, fat, skinny, bald (yes, I know I said it once already) you are. Tough noogies. (Again, not the term I would normally use.) I'm not recommending that you whine all the time. In fact, please don't or you'll give this book a bad reputation, but if anyone tells you to stop talking about it, I suggest you take into consideration that your illness may frighten or burden them. And then, after you consider that, tell them

you need them to be more supportive. Remember—you have cancer! Yes, I went there. I tried several alternatives. Being frank and open about what you need is, in my opinion, the best way to go.

5. When people start to tell you their horror stories of family or people they know who had one form of cancer or another, stop them in midsentence. Really! Do not listen, or else later you may not be able to tune out their voices in your head. Stop them right in the middle, and just say, "Thank you, but I really find it too difficult to listen to stories like that." Period. I know it's impossible to imagine saying that, but I'm here to tell you—this is important. You're the one who will lie awake in the middle of the night unable to shake that story from your mind. You do not need to take that on. Self-protection is hugely important for this period in your life.

That's a lot about "normal" in terms of how you feel and might respond to others. But that's only the half of it. Because, of course, we can't talk about "normal" without talking about how you look.

DEALING WITH YOUR SELF-IMAGE

There is no way to prepare for the effect that all this trauma has on your self-image. I don't think it matters whether you are vain or relatively low maintenance when it comes to your looks. I thought I was low maintenance. I rarely wore makeup and didn't spend that much time, money, or effort putting myself together on a daily basis. I mean, I knew how to put it on when it was important, but I wasn't focused on looking in the mirror or getting up early every day to do my hair and makeup. So I thought I could handle it. I thought I could just power through. Boy, was I wrong! The physical changes of a mastectomy and chemotherapy are just so dramatic that everyone I've spoken to had big issues with them. Your face without hair is hard to recognize; your body post-surgery is hard to recognize. Put that together with the daily question marks of how you feel and what it all means, and it can be a recipe for major meltdowns. Notice the plural.

I don't know anyone who sailed through the treatment and surgery without taking a temporary self-image hit. You know it's coming, you prepare yourself as best you can, but it's still tricky to look in the mirror some days.

TOP 5 TIPS FOR DEALING
WITH YOUR SELF-IMAGE

∽

1. Don't be embarrassed to seek emotional and psychological help. Dealing with your self-image is a
huge part of healing, and most cancer patients can
get enormous benefits talking with people outside their inner circle. It takes a *looooooong* time
to work through it all, and your friends and family
can only understand so much. They really want and
need you to focus on your fight, your success, and
your life, but you need to have time to process the
rest. And it should take . . . well, as long as it takes.

2. There are many ways to find the help you need. Try
a support group if you're a group person. In fact,
try a support group even if you're not a group person. And try another one if you don't like the first
one. There is no substitute for being with people
who've gone through all this themselves. Not even
this book.

3. Find a therapist who specializes in cancer patients—
your oncologist can recommend one—and go. Your
local American Cancer Society chapter may have

one on staff. Going even once or twice might help you decide if you need more. It's a very alien feeling to get up bald, newly thin or fat, or no eyelashes or eyebrows, put on a wig, then makeup, then a prosthetic breast—get it all together so you look a little bit like your former self—and then have people tell you how fabulous, or tired, or terrific, or exhausted you look. It can feel a little like being a clown in the circus. Of course it's the most messed-up circus ever, not the sparkly and magical Cirque du Soleil kind. Sometimes you just have to slap on the clown makeup and costume and go out there.

4. Bald really *is* better with earrings. There's something about adding a little femininity to a masculine picture. Seriously, flat chest, bald head—I started to look like my grandfather; though lovely, not a handsome man! So wear some jewelry.

5. Look at yourself. I'm serious. Try really hard not to shy away from mirrors, even if the reflection is more fun house than fun. Eventually you will see that it really is you in there, and that's what others see, too. The real you doesn't need hair or breasts to be beautiful. It's still your eyes and your smile. Sometimes it just takes practice to see it.

DEALING WITH OTHERS' IMAGES OF YOU

People will say the most outrageous things to you—and especially shocking things about the way you look. One of my poor friends was told she looked like a poodle, Rod Stewart, and some butch (no offense) woman from the gym. They'll say you look great, tired, can carry off that scarf/hat, too skinny, bloated, pretty, just like yourself (who else would you look like? Rod Stewart?).

Most want so much for you not to focus on the negative that they'll say anything to try to help. Sadly it never does. My poor mother, who'd been an absolute angel through my whole process, just didn't know what to say to help me feel better about how I looked. Every time she saw me, she'd tell me how beautiful I looked or how good my hair looked. No matter what she said, it was the wrong thing. I finally told her to please stop talking about my hair or how I looked. I knew it was coming from the heart, but I just couldn't take it. I think any mention of how you look, whether compliment or insult, reminds you of how you actually look. My husband told me I looked like a beautiful alien. Hmmm, I know he meant well, but I kept picturing those guys with the smooth green skin and huge eyes.

No matter what people say, it will probably provoke some sort of internal reaction in you. If they say you look fabulous, you may think: If they'd only seen me an hour ago, bald and naked! If they say you look tired, you may think: I spent this entire time getting ready, thought I looked great, and I still look tired? No matter what, I'm never going to look like my old self. These feelings are common, and they can lead to a more serious kind of detachment from your self-image, so it is helpful to find professionals whom you can trust. Otherwise the feelings can lead to the same kinds of perceptions anorexics have when they look in the mirror, see someone looking back who weighs eighty pounds, and think they're fat. Your brain can do weird things to your psyche, even if you've never had body issues before. And who knows a woman without body issues?

This is what support groups and therapists are good for. I may be overstating it, but if you want to find real understanding, I think it's impossible to talk to anyone other than someone who has gone through this or who specializes in it.

9

Sex, Drugs, and No More Rock and Roll

The day I was diagnosed with breast cancer, I was advised to start taking antianxiety medication to help with sleep and other issues during the day. Every woman I spoke to was given similar advice. I took it. It didn't really help me sleep, so my oncologist and I played with a few medications, trying to settle into something that would get me at least five or six hours of sleep a night so I didn't get psychotic. In the meantime I started A/C treatments, which meant new meds for hot flashes caused by the drugs and induced menopause, and then even more drugs for sleeping. Everything started out just fine, and my doctors figured out a combination that helped me sleep better than I had in years. The only problem was that I was slowly starting to feel like I was losing my mind. We get so focused on the physical side effects of all the drugs, it's easy to overlook the mental and behavioral ones that are also listed and are no less real. Emotional and behavioral side effects are actually the result of chemical changes in the brain, physical changes that simply show up as changed behaviors or emotions. It's really easy to forget that and to assume your feelings or reactions to things are not worth mentioning to your doctor. You may experience behavioral or mood changes that are easily swept under the rug of stress, but really they could be drug reactions and side effects, so don't underestimate them.

TOP 5 TIPS FOR HANDLING ALL THE MEDICATIONS

1. Make sure you read all the side effects listed in the information provided with every drug, and give them all equal weight.

2. Make sure you check with your oncologist before adding any new drugs to those you already take. Antibiotics, herbal supplements—yes, hair-growth vitamins and other "natural" or "organic" remedies are actually drugs—you get the idea. This is not the time to self-medicate or to trust that your local pharmacist has checked all possible drug

interactions. In your appointments you will most likely be asked if you made any changes to your medications; just make sure you include any supplements.

3. Talk to your doctor. In the beginning (following surgery and at the start of chemo) it is super important to take all the drugs your doctor recommends, but there may come a point later on where you want to start weaning off some of the medications. Remember when I said I thought I was losing my mind? I kind of was. I was on so many pills I didn't know which way was up. I felt like I could be arrested for the amount of stuff in my body. I finally told my doctor I wanted to get off anything that wasn't saving my life. As she made clear, you can't just go cold turkey; you have to have a plan. Over a period of a month or two, we dropped a whole series of drugs I'd been taking. Then we added back the things I really needed to feel better and combat symptoms.

4. Read and reread the labels to make sure you take the prescribed drugs in the prescribed amounts. This is a good time to reiterate the suggestion that you write the drugs' names and doses on top of all

your medicine bottles, so you can easily identify what's what. At one point I was taking more than thirty-six pills a day!

5. Take your medicine. Time to be a big girl. Even though you may get sick of—and from—treatments, do it anyway. Skipping it or refusing treatment will just make it worse. I was truly surprised to hear that some people stop in the middle of treatments, or skip some because of how it makes them feel. Stay with it! It may be saving your life.

And you thought I was going to talk about sex....

SEX

For many people this is a tricky, delicate subject, even before all the added benefits of diagnosis, surgery, pain, body-image issues, drugs, side effects, etc. So imagine what the effects of everything that's happening to you might be. Remember, your body not only feels different, it actually *is* different every day. This means you may respond unexpectedly to stimuli and actions you're used to trusting. The blood flow to your erogenous zones is different during chemo. Some people find it very difficult to reach orgasm during treatment. I'm not going to tell you personal stories about this, but don't assume (or let your partner assume) that your reactions are simply emotional responses. They may very well be physical, and something that doesn't work one day may work perfectly well the next, or at a different time of day. Or maybe it's time to try new things.

Try to consider this an opportunity to throw away the old playbook and write a new one. Think about it. If your taste buds are different all the time, maybe you need to adjust your tastes. Get it? Personally, the lack of pubic hair was a revelation. Literally and figuratively!

TOP 5 TIPS FOR SEX AND THE NEW YOU

∞

1. Keep your expectations low. Your body has been thrown into turmoil, and both your sex drive and your physiological responses are going to be out of whack.

---

2. Don't take whatever happens too seriously. This is not how things will be forever. Try just to go with the flow. If you feel sexy one day, go for it, but don't be distressed if those moments are few and far between.

3. Do not be alarmed if your partner doesn't seem interested. It may be too difficult to see you as a patient one day and a sex object the next. Don't take it personally. Just because you can switch gears one day doesn't mean he can, too. It won't mean that he doesn't find you attractive anymore—it may just mean that he's in caregiver mode.

4. Use birth control. (And if you're on the pill, tell your doctor; remember, it's yet another drug you're adding to the chemical cauldron in your body.) It's possible to get pregnant during chemotherapy, but it's not a good idea. Your hormones will be very unbalanced for the whole process and for up to a year or so after; you may be fertile without realizing it.

5. Use a non-petroleum-based lubricant. Chemo interferes with many bodily functions, including lubrication. Medically induced menopause can cause dryness, so you need to protect the tissues.

PARTNERS AND CAREGIVERS

Okay, so this is a loaded gun. My husband and I went through a lot from the day I was diagnosed. As we found out, that's entirely normal. Your friends and doctors (and I) will tell you over and over how important it is for you to focus on yourself and your needs. And you're bound to feel so overwhelmed that you really do need their permission to do just that. You can no longer do everything you used to, and you will have to depend on others to help out. However, you will also come to realize that your partner, family, and caregivers have needs, too. (How very annoying of them to have needs while you have cancer!) Working out accommodations for their needs is a crucial part of the process.

TOP 5 TIPS FOR
HELPING YOUR CAREGIVER

1. Encourage your caregiver to seek professional help during this time. Today's cancer professionals have realized how important caregivers are and how challenging it is to be one. Most towns and cities

have caregiver support groups. Help your caregiver find them.

2. Encourage him or her to take breaks, go out with friends, take a few days off. These next months are all about you, but if your caregiver is too drained or too isolated, that affects both your partnership and your well-being. My poor husband finally took a few days for himself with a friend, only to have his father pass away during his trip. No break for him! Plus, when we got home, I was way too wrapped up in my own issues to give him enough support. Poor guy. I still feel awful about that time in our lives.

3. Take some time every once in a while to appreciate what's being done for you. Even if you think there are lots of holes in what is being done. The fact is that those in your family are the only ones dealing with you every day and night, and regardless of how well or badly they are handling it, they deserve credit for handling it at all. It sucks. Gratefully accept the help you are being given, and please, please ask (nicely) for what you're not getting and still need. Nobody's perfect, and there's no manual for how to be the perfect caregiver. I told my

husband he should write one (he's the real writer in the family), and he just laughed.

4. Don't forget that your partner's life has been thrown into turmoil, too, and there's lots of fear involved. My husband walked around for the first few months saying that he couldn't access his feelings. Well, that didn't help me at all. He just couldn't deal right away with his fear of the diagnosis and its consequences, so whenever I tried to talk about my own fears, he would just tell me I was going to be fine. Lots of people do this. They can't bear to hear you being afraid, when all you really need to do is to be able to say it out loud and have him respond, "I know you're scared. How can you not be?"

5. Occasionally go to the doctor without anyone else. I know that all the literature (including this book) says that you should always have someone with you, but every once in a while, I felt the need to go by myself to my doctor's appointments. Sometimes there are questions you don't want to ask in front of anyone else. It's a good idea to bring a notebook or use your smartphone to record the appointment so you can remember what is said—but sometimes it's good for everyone to be alone.

It's also really important to do things together that are not doctor or disease related. It's really difficult to do, but it feels so good to try to forget for a while. Treating cancer becomes your partnership's full-time job, and sometimes you both need a vacation.

NO MORE ROCK AND ROLL

There are days when you feel relatively normal during treatment. You'll feel a lot like your old self, going about your old life. Then something might happen to bring you up short and remind you that it wasn't a bad dream, that you do live on the other side of the street now.

One day I was running errands for my son, picking up his contact lenses at the optometrist's office in a major hospital complex. I walked into the elevator having forgotten which floor the office was on. I stared at the buttons and wondered out loud, "Okay, which floor am I going to?" The man next to me said, "Oncology? Second floor." *Wham!* Back to reality. That was how people saw me. Even when you go about your normal life, and you feel like a regular person, somebody may bring you crashing back. That's me—Cancer Girl. Sort of like the exact opposite of

Wonder Woman. Cancer Girl is the one who wears the scarf and didn't have time or energy to put on all the makeup that hides her lack of eyelashes. Cancer Girl is the one with the really pale skin and breaking fingernails. She's the one who is so tired she's in bed by seven p.m. on most nights.

When you are feeling relatively normal, it's really hard to be pulled back into cancerland. Sometimes all it takes is a loved one reaching out and saying, with that concern in their eyes, "How are you?" It's just such a loaded question. Half the time you want to say "Fine," because how else can you answer? I mean, honestly, you could list all your side effects and fears and lack of sleep. Or whip off your wig and say, "How do you *think* I feel?" Or jump up and down with joy that there are only two chemo treatments left or that your latest scan showed a shrinking tumor. At this point in my journey (I really hate that word; I'd say this experience was more like an arctic trek on foot—with no shoes), I found the only time that question had the right feel was when my dad asked me, because he had been diagnosed with early-stage lung cancer just a few years before, and so he "got it." He continues to get it—that C-word that exists in a cartoon bubble over your head now, but that you refuse to let define you.

TOP 1 TIP FOR DEALING
WITH CANCER GIRL

∽

There's really only one good tip for dealing with this:

1. Find a support group. I've mentioned this before, but it bears repeating here. Talking to people who've been where you are is more helpful emotionally than anything else. Especially if you are one of those women who doesn't want anyone to feel sorry for you. (Personally I enjoy a little sympathy every now and then. Especially if it comes with chocolate.) It's critically important to find a safe place where you feel free to express your concerns and fears and where they won't be taken out of context or perceived as weakness.

10

The End of Treatment

Maybe you have a day circled on your calendar. The last day of chemo. The last day of radiation. Personally I could never keep track of when everything was supposed to end. Lots of women I spoke to had the same issue. Everyone wants to know when you're done, but it's hard to keep it locked in your mind. Maybe because things keep changing, or maybe because it seems like it will never end, so that a single day on the calendar didn't seem to mean as much to me as it did to everyone around me.

On the last day of radiation, which for me was the last day of external treatments (I still take oral medications daily), my husband and parents came to the session. In the last week of treatments everyone kept saying, "You're almost done! Don't you feel great? Aren't you excited?" I didn't and I wasn't. But I wasn't totally surprised. My therapist had warned me (as had some wonderful women who had gone through the same thing) that the end of treatment is a very bizarre feeling for many women.

One of my friends said she felt as though she wasn't fighting anymore, and she hated that feeling. Studies show that it is not until after the end of treatment that many people really start to feel what has happened to them. Up until that point we are so bombarded with information and physically assaulted by treatment that the mind can't process everything. You're just in survival mode.

That's not to say that along the way you don't wake up and wonder what the heck happened to you, or feel crushed by anxiety or fear. But often the full cognitive awareness of everything you've gone through starts to kick in when treatment is finished. All of a sudden your brain has time to react instead of just focusing on the fight, the next dose of poison, and the doctors' appointments. So, on that last day of radiation, while my mother cried from relief in the waiting room, and my husband shook his fists in a victory salute, and everyone called to congratulate me, I knew my family and friends wanted me to feel like one of those wind-up monkeys banging cymbals together. But I couldn't. I felt nothing. Well, maybe not nothing. I was relieved not to have to go to the hospital every single day. I was relieved not to feel like a bag of microwave popcorn anymore. I was relieved that nothing new was going to be done to my body for a while.

I did all the things you're supposed to do at the end of treatment. I made my famous chocolate cookies for the staff and smiled at everyone who said, "Congratulations, you're done!" But I didn't feel it. I felt hollow. First of all, I knew that the true effects of the radiation had yet to appear. And even though I was feeling oh-so superior because of how well my skin was holding up, I knew there was more pain to come.

On top of all that was the fear that I wasn't done. Sure, I had made it through surgery, chemotherapy, and radiation. I had lost a breast, my hair, fingernails, skin, my work, and almost a year of my life. I had made it through all that, but I couldn't shake the feeling that I wasn't done. What if it came back? Could I go through all this again?

The next day, however, I woke up feeling a whole lot lighter. Simply not having to go to the hospital turned out to be a huge weight off my mind. Sometimes you don't realize what a drain something is until it's gone.

My husband and I decided to take a trip about three weeks after the end of my radiation. I was so worried about how I would feel that it was hard for me to get excited, but when the day came, I really felt quite well. By then my skin had started to heal, the pain was mostly gone, and I'd started to feel like a human being again. Even my eyelashes were back. Getting out of town, away from anything that remotely reminded either of us of the horrible time we'd just gone through, was great healing for my mind as well. Sure, I still didn't have my energy back. Sure, I still had to dress in flowing tops and scarves, because I had one breast and was still too raw from radiation to wear a bra. Sure, my hair was so short that it was barely covering my whole head and was a peculiar shade of tan, but at least I was away from the hospitals, doctors, sad eyes, and polite smiles of cancer. I could just be with my husband and be me. Hot-flashing, pale, relatively sleepless, afternoon-napping, but happy to be done and praying for a long future—me.

CHEMO BRAIN

I have to admit—I assumed chemo brain was a myth. Well, maybe not a complete myth, but I thought it probably had something to do with just being tired of the whole process. I didn't actually think about it as a long-lasting side effect. That is, until it hit *me*. I started to have word-retrieval issues, difficulty finding the word I wanted to say. Or I'd use the wrong word when talking. Or have trouble pronouncing words. I even stuttered. My family teased me in the beginning, the way you would anyone making a Freudian slip. Except that these moments were not Freudian, they were freaky! When they realized what was behind my issues, they were kinder. But I felt stupid—often. Not a feeling I relished.

One other strange thing that I didn't realize had anything to do with chemo, but it does: I couldn't multitask for a while. If I was doing something, and people started to talk to me or ask me questions, I would get anxious. I'd lose my place, either in whatever I was doing or in the conversation. It was a terribly unsettling feeling. The anxiety made me irritable in those moments. Oddly, my doctors—as good and conscientious as they were—had glossed over chemo brain. They'd mentioned it, but only in passing, and I hadn't really focused on it. And then there it was: full-blown symptoms.

My therapist—bless her—explained that all these problems were actually documented side effects of chemotherapy. Something about how the chemicals continue to affect your brain for some time after you've completed the therapy. The symptoms are temporary, but can last up to—and even longer than—a year. Within a few months of finishing radiation, I began to see real improvement, but I was certainly not back to normal. It takes a while.

Advice: More of the same: No matter what physical or psychological symptoms you're feeling, if something seems odd and new and worrisome to you, talk to your doctor. And don't be afraid to make it absolutely clear how much the symptoms are bothering you. Not everybody responds the same way to cancer treatments, and it's your body. You're the one who actually knows what's happening. Chances are you're experiencing some sort of side effect. Even if your doctor can't do anything to make it better, it helps to know you're not crazy! If your doctor is unsympathetic, find someone who has loads of experience with cancer patients to talk to.

CONTINUING TREATMENTS

There are many continuing treatments for breast cancer, both oral medications and infusions. You may have Herceptin infusions on a regular basis or be on Tamoxifen. You may, like me, have bisphosphonate infusions (like Zometa) or any number of other medications. None of these ongoing preventive measures should include the level of side effects that you experienced with chemotherapy. Your hair will grow back, your energy will gradually increase, and you will start to feel like yourself again. Mostly. And you will begin to feel like you can move on from just being in survival mode.

In the first two years after my diagnosis, I felt slightly uncomfortable with new people until I knew that they knew what had happened to me. I considered it too huge an event in my life for them not to know about it if we were going to have any kind of real friendship. But it's not the kind of thing you mention when you meet someone, so it's a little awkward at first. I suppose if you're a really private person, this won't bother you—we rarely know what others have truly gone through in their lives—but I did feel that the physical and emotional changes were so protracted, so profound, that it was necessary for me to find a way to tell almost everyone. Writing this book was a good introduction for me, because when new people asked me what I did, I could say I was writing a book. Invariably they'd ask me the topic and— voilà—ice breaker. Well, more like the *Titanic*, but at least it was out there.

Of course not everyone feels this way. I know many women who prefer to put the whole experience behind them and move forward as if it never happened. They don't want to have people see them as sick or weak. That's okay, too. Regardless of your personal perception, the fact is that you will have *some* sort of feeling about it. Like it or not (and nobody likes it), it's now a part of who you are, and that stupid elephant with its big lumbering feet and "Breast Cancer Awareness" button on its trunk is standing right next to you every day.

SCAR TISSUE—THE EMOTIONAL KIND

Anyone who has had any kind of cancer knows that the scar tissue from the diagnosis and treatment is more than skin deep. A cigar is never just a cigar. Every ache and pain is either a reminder of the past or a harbinger of evil in your future. A wonderful support volunteer at the Breast Cancer Resource Center of Santa Barbara told me that fifteen years after her diagnosis, she had a chronic pain in her toe and went to see her oncologist, fearing a recurrence. Her doctor reassured her that people really don't get cancer of the toe, but I empathized completely. It's out there. You now know that your body is capable of turning against you, and you can't help wondering when it will happen again.

After being told for all these months to be hypersensitive to your body and all its reactions, now you're suddenly supposed to turn it off and go back to ignoring pains in your toes. Guess what? Not going to happen right away. You've got to retrain yourself, and it takes a while. Once you've crossed the street, you're stuck on this side forever. It's not so easy for your caregivers on the other side, either. They can't imagine what the big deal is over every little ache and pain, or they've been retrained, too, and now they won't even let you move a chair. There it is again, the "new normal."

Nevertheless you can't let the fear paralyze you. It gets easier over time to forget for a while and just live from scan to scan. In the beginning, though, what kept me up at night was not the fear of dying, but the fear of having to live through it all again. I just had to tell myself that at that moment in time, I was cancer-free and should live that way.

Around this time I also found myself starting to get a false sense of control about what the future might hold. Breast cancer treatments come with a constant flow of advice and directives, and it all sounds so positive. I had all these medications and treatment plans and vitamins and exercises and tests, and I started to develop a belief that if I just did everything right, everything carefully, this thing would really be under my control. I had to remind myself that the fact is it's not. I didn't cause it, and I can't control whether it comes back. All I can do is follow the plan my doctors set out for me.

So when your partner says (because he has to, for himself), "You're going to beat this. You're strong. You're going to be fine," sometimes that's hard to take. The truth is, you have no idea. If it comes back it's not your fault; it doesn't mean you were weak or didn't try hard enough. It's a disease that we just don't know enough about. So don't be angry at him, but do make sure he knows how it makes you feel. And don't forget to tell him how great he is for the little things he does—even for just sticking around—because some people can't handle it all and run for the hills.

WHY DOESN'T HE CALL?
WAITING FOR RESULTS

One of the hardest things to live with is the fear of recurrence. Even in this book, it's a recurring theme. For the first year after treatment you will probably have scans every three months. Eventually they'll move to every six months, and then nine, and then a year. It seems to be a universal experience that about a week before a scan, anxiety sets in. How can it not? It's natural to be afraid. The thing is, though, that fear can warp your sense of reality. Lots of people (myself included) interpret that anxiety as a bad feeling that something is wrong. Then when something does go wrong, you get to say, "I knew it. I had a bad feeling." Of course when everything's fine, you forget that you drove yourself, and probably everyone around you, crazy.

When I went for one of my first follow-ups, I was getting off the table after the PET/CT scan had been completed, and the nurse said to me, "The radiologist would like to take some more pictures with one of the other machines." I almost passed out. My knees got wobbly, and my heart started beating so fast I thought I was going to have a heart attack. She led me to a chair and left to prepare the digital mammogram machine. My heart skipped more than a beat. It ran all the way back one year. I had to sit on that little chair outside the room and wait. And wait. In the hours (okay, six minutes) that it took for the nurse to come back, I ran about a million (okay, five) scenarios in my head. I just sat there trying to calm myself down. I was alone in the examining area, with my parents sitting out in the waiting room reading *House Beautiful* and *Sports Illustrated*. I imagined having to come out and tell them. I imagined calling my husband to come home from work. How would my son, away at prep school, deal with this from so many miles away? How would my daughter live through another round of Steroid Mommy? In those few minutes I went through it all again in my head. My hair! Not again!

Then I was led back into the room and placed in the familiar position. You know, the one between the plastic torture trays. Only this time I was sitting. The nurse told me to stay still for—get this—twelve minutes! I kid you not. Twelve minutes. In those twelve minutes I had more than enough time to contemplate my fate. I ran through all the very good reasons I had chosen not to have a prophylactic mastectomy on that side. I thought they were good reasons at the time, but now, sitting flattened and in pain, they seemed absurd. Then the nurse returned and released my pancake. Pause and reset. This time I had the presence of mind to tell her that I hadn't eaten or had anything to drink all day, and I was about ready to pass out. I left out the part where I thought my heart was going to jump out of my chest, because I figured when it did, they'd be able to see it on the mammogram. She brought me a little cup of water. She held my breast hostage while I sipped.

When my boob and I were finally released, I had

to go home and wait for the results. Of course I was given no information at the follow-up, and we had two days before we could see my oncologist because it was Friday afternoon. Note to self—do not go for tests on Fridays! I didn't say anything to my parents, just that it took longer than expected. When my husband came home, he tried his best to be reassuring, but I know he must have been terrified. Then, after a sleepless weekend, we went to see my oncologist. He was, of course, running exceptionally late, having been dealing with some emergency. Finally he came in the door and said everything was fine. We were so relieved and clearly more upset than he'd anticipated. I said I was so nervous because of the extra tests. He said, "Oh, that was nothing. The radiologist just couldn't see your breast well enough from the other position." *What*? Are you kidding me? That's it? They put me through that anxiety, cortisol running through my body, my husband and I convincing ourselves that we could handle whatever happened, for nothing? Next time, how about the radiologist coming out and telling the patient that little tidbit, instead of, "The doctor would like more pictures"?!

So, for the record, don't make any assumptions. You may be completely misinterpreting the need for more pictures, another test, whatever. A year earlier

I'd had an MRI, and they called me to come back the next day because the tech had done the test wrong and not taken the right pictures. I swear that's what they said. I called my brother, the radiologist, to ask if that was likely, because I was convinced they were lying just to get me back in for more tests after they'd seen something else.

The cold, hard truth is that the anxiety is going to be with you for life. Meet it head-on, but don't let it morph out of control. First of all remember what I said before—that results are rarely cut and dried. There's often a hitch. Either they want more pictures, or some number is just a little off—any number of things can obscure the results. Your body is incredibly complex, and now everyone's on high alert. It's an early-warning system, and sometimes you have to hold tight while they figure out that the blip on the radar screen is just a bird, not an incoming fighter jet.

Because I moved from Seattle to California, I've had experiences with two separate oncologists, and they handled results in exactly the same way. So, in this very scientific study of mine, the conclusions are clear: Doctors do not like to call their patients with good news. Or bad news, for that matter. They prefer to have you wait for your scheduled appointment, because that way you're not reading something into every minute that passes. Though it's hard to imagine, all the good doctors have lots and lots of patients, and sometimes they're focused on other people (what nerve!) and can't call. And then you're in a puddle on your kitchen floor, convinced you're dying.

Forget the cancer; that afternoon in the digital mammogram took ten years off my life. And that's the day I learned to try not to make assumptions. The truth may be that you were at a funny angle in the machine, or you took a deep breath, or they want the same exact view as last time. It's not always because there's something there. The trick is to remind yourself of this. *Every time.* Of course I still want to go back in and kill that radiologist, and maybe hold the nurse hostage for twelve minutes while I'm at it.

LOOKING FORWARD

Right after my treatment had ended, I got seven months of my life back. It turns out that the doctors start counting your healthy days from the day of diagnosis. I always thought it was from the last day of treatment. Neat trick, huh? So when you've had your second scan in six months, after six months of treatment, you're really a year out! That was the day I found out I was a two-year cancer-free survivor. It's details like that that seem to get lost in the shuffle. So you get to be a survivor counting from the day your life fell apart.

OCTOBER

October is the toughest month. It is a wonderful thing for the future of breast cancer treatment and diagnosis to have so much attention focused on breast cancer awareness. But I will tell you that, as a survivor, it's really rough. Everyone I know dreads the sudden appearance of pink ribbons, pink labels on yogurt, and even the pink cleats and towels on the NFL players. The preponderance of TV movies, *Today* show specials, and newly released films with the funny and brave woman fighting her battle while looking decidedly upbeat in her festive silk scarf sends me running for the hills. Every time I see an actress playing bald on TV, it bugs me that they don't shave or pluck her eyebrows. I mean, come on, make an effort! Also, a scarf looks decidedly different on a head that is actually bald than when it's covering hair. And I'm always looking for that shadow that the tiny hairs make around the ears and back of the neck, the telltale sign of a full head of hair.

Being asked by the grocery store clerk whether I'd

like to donate to breast cancer awareness brings up a sudden urge to pull up my shirt, show off my scar, and yell, "No, thanks! I'm *already aware!*"

Expect to have very mixed feelings during the entire month. On the one hand, participating in one of the walks for the cure was one of the most gratifying and emotional experiences of my life. I walked with my family and a friend, and there was something very powerful about being surrounded by pink shirts and hats and bald women, all smiling and cheering. Crossing the finish line and into the lane for survivors, where they placed a medal around my neck, truly felt like winning an Olympic medal.

On the other hand, the T-shirts and posters commemorating lost mothers, sisters, and friends were a constant reminder of my uncertain future. Walking behind five women wearing T-shirts with a photograph of a smiling woman and her dates of life and death was like following one of the ghosts in *A Christmas Carol*. I had to find a spot with real live people and no photographs.

The month of October is thirty-one days filled with constant reminders that you are going to be one of those women crossing the finish line in the survivors' lane. Even if you don't participate in any organized breast cancer awareness activity, the pink tsunami will bring up every thought and feeling you've ever had, plus a few more. Don't be surprised by this, and don't expect it to change over time. Women I know who are fifteen years out still feel the same way. I encourage you to embrace the part of it that helps you realize you are not alone. There is strength to be gained during this month by the sheer number of people who share your journey. Walk with them, run with them, cheer with them, talk with them, cry with them. It will help. Then, before you know it, you can dress up for Halloween and start thinking about Thanksgiving and other holidays that don't involve chemo. Personally I'm thinking of dressing up as a giant boob (just one), but I can't figure out how to sew that costume.

FEAR OF DYING

Obviously this is a huge issue from the moment you are called back for more pictures during your mammogram. In the very beginning there is so much to do and go through that it almost gets swept under the rug of doctors' appointments, surgery, staging, and treatment. It is more than an elephant in the room. It's a herd of elephants in your head, heart, and mind. It is the subtitle of the book called breast cancer. It is always there and can influence your attitude and behaviors in ways you don't realize or imagine unless you take those elephants out for a walk once in a while.

Talking about it with family and friends who had not gone through anything like this was very unsatisfying to me. Those people can only tell you that it will be okay. You will be fine. You are young, strong, and so on. You have great doctors, and you're going to beat it. Blah, blah, blah. For me, at least, it did not help. The fear is real. It's in the statistics. It's in the stories that say, "After a fourteen-year battle with breast cancer . . ." It's in the word "spread." It's in the waiting room at the doctor's office. It's there before every follow-up scan. It's in your head. You have to give voice to it. Seeing a therapist who specializes in cancer patients is a good way to do this. Or a support group at the hospital or breast cancer center. Or a local chapter of Gilda's Club. Keep trying different ways of handling the fear and feelings, and don't give up until you find an outlet that's right for you. It's out there.

I don't want to get all new-agey now, but there are lessons to be learned from going through this horrible experience. Many women, including me, learned to accept help. We learned that being sick is not being weak. We learned to be humble in the face of our bodies. We learned to be our own advocates. We learned to feel pretty in spite of the mirror. We learned the importance of slowing down. We learned who our friends are. We learned we can help others with our support and our stories.

There are lots of life-affirming things you can do. I wrote this book.

TOP 5 TIPS FOR GETTING ON WITH YOUR LIFE

1. Forgive and forget. Try your level best not to play the blame game. This can be super difficult when you live in a world where you are constantly bombarded with cancer prevention strategies. I was plagued by questions like: Did I eat too much sugar? Not exercise enough? Should I be a vegan now? All that. Whatever the cause of your initial cancer, there's nothing you can do about it now. It's in the past, and it's time to focus on your future—because you have one. Follow your doctor's orders. Make lifestyle changes if they're warranted, and don't beat yourself up about how you got here.

---

2. Stay vigilant but enjoy yourself, too. As I mentioned, hypervigilance is a natural response to what you've been through. It's normal to be extra sensitive to every new ache and pain and wonder if it's cancer. Voice your fears to your support network and doctors, and when they tell you it's okay, really try to focus on that. There are plenty of nerve-racking moments ahead (like the night before a scan) so try to push those thoughts aside when they come out so you don't let them overwhelm the good days.

3. Don't be surprised when Cancer Girl makes an appearance. Life after diagnosis is a complicated, ever-changing patchwork of emotions. For weeks on end that pink elephant just stands quietly in a corner and doesn't draw my attention, and then suddenly, seemingly without warning, *cancer* is all I can think about. This is normal. Sometimes the happiness at my survival far outweighs the fear of recurrence and the physical changes the disease has forced on my body. Other times the scars and fears are front and center. When that happens, the best thing to do is talk it out. Face that elephant and make it go back in the corner.

4. The feeling of being in limbo will go away. In the first one to three years right after treatment, many patients feel a sense of uncertainty, hovering between being well and being a patient. You're still adapting to the many physical and emotional changes of the past months, and just because treatment is over, it doesn't mean you feel like a survivor. You essentially have PTSD, so give it time. When I say "time" I mean months, even a year. Not a few weeks.

5. Just get on with it already. If only it were that easy. This is exactly how your friends and family may want you to feel after a while. It may be exactly how *you* want to feel after a while. You do not need to let cancer define the rest of your life the way it has defined this part of your life. I never say there's life after cancer, because I never feel there is an "after cancer." There *is* life after diagnosis and life after treatment, though. So:

Go out and live it!

ACKNOWLEDGMENTS

I gratefully acknowledge the incredible medical staff at Swedish Hospital in Seattle: all of my doctors and nurses who gave me the tools to fight and the advice that has found its way into every page of this book. In particular:

Erin Ellis, MD, medical oncologist, Swedish Hospital, who was there from the very beginning.

Mikul Gupta, MD, medical oncologist/hematologist, Samsun Clinic, who continues to provide me with the best care I could hope for.

Thank you to my editor and publisher, Karen Rinaldi, for believing this book could be a help to women, and for her expert guidance.

And my agent, Sandy Dijkstra, for helping this book become a reality.

ABOUT THE AUTHOR

A graduate of Duke University and an interior designer, Andrea Hutton was diagnosed with breast cancer in 2009 at the age of forty-one. Andrea is now five years out and cancer-free. In addition to continuing her interior design career for select clients, Andrea is a marketing and management consultant. She lives in Santa Barbara, California, with her husband and two children.